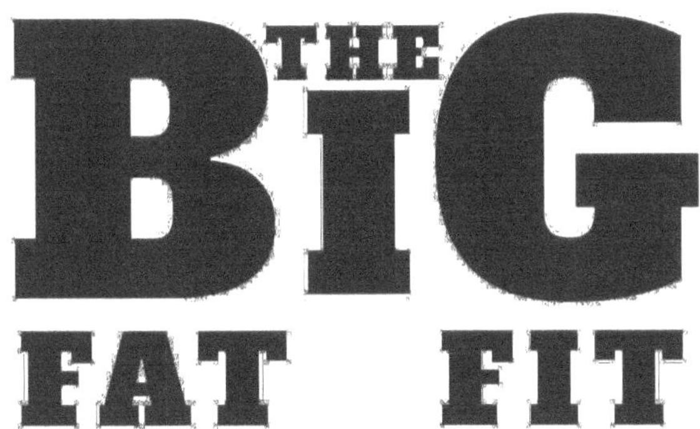

SECRETS OF EATING AND DRINKING ANYTHING AND STILL BEING THE FITTEST PERSON IN YOUR CIRCLE!

BY CHIRAG BHARADWAJ

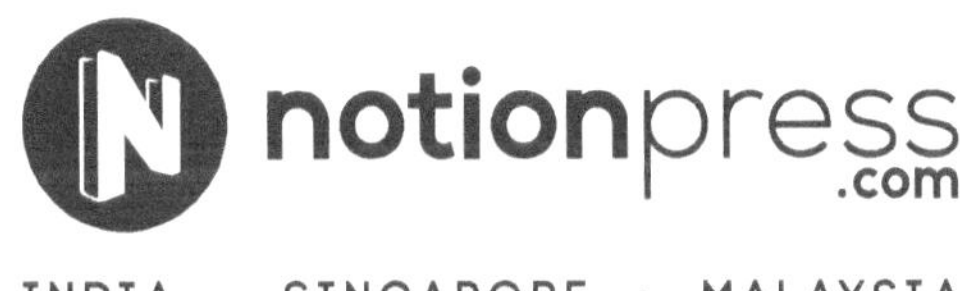

Notion Press

No.8, 3rd Cross Street
CIT Colony, Mylapore
Chennai, Tamil Nadu – 600004

First Published by Notion Press 2020
Copyright © Chirag Bharadwaj 2020
All Rights Reserved.

ISBN: 978-1-63745-352-0

CONTENTS

PREFACE

Everybody wants freedom. In some way or the other, we all want to feel liberated. Freedom for me is simply, unboundedness, independence, and free will. Let's call it "doing what you want, whenever you want to". Freedom can be sought in many aspects of life. All I sought for a huge chunk of my short life was freedom from 2 things. Food, Exercise. Or as I call, nutritional and fitness freedom. I was in a cage not many of you are unaware of. Key word, WAS. Freedom is also why I am writing this book. Freedom from all the questions, doubts, asking of my opinion and 100 other things by scores of people in my life and on the internet. Also, this is aimed to provide the very same freedom, to you, the reader that picked up this book. I believe it was not morally right to give the same truncated answers every time nor was it long-term sustainable for me to keep giving this "expert opinion" till I die. By writing this book, I transfer the power to whom it should always belong, you.

In the age of technology, apps, influencers and quick internet fixes to your problems, especially fitness problems, the average baby boomer and millennial is headed into a state of degeneracy. This is because eating and being fit are external, physical, real life practices. Much beyond what an article or a social media post or an app can fix. Having faced it first hand, writing this was a no brainer.

I believe I have done everything to tell my story from fat to fit (less important) and project my belief on this topic. Articles, Videos, Social Media, etc and now this book. I have dragged myself through it all, more than half of my (short) life spent erring, learning, improving and trying to perfect this part of life.

I can now say that it is on autopilot. This fitness thing is a healthy hobby and an essential part of my life you know, not by any means a profession.

Which is precisely why a view, like mine, someone who is not a "personal trainer" or a "dietician" is a gold mine for you. I have nothing but veracity to provide.

Information will never cease to exist, that is something that I want you to explore by your own volition. But what I have come to understand is that this is a highly obfuscated field, especially for an outsider, like I was once. I thought only a meticulously written piece of literature, that I majorly wrote during the months and weeks leading up to and during COVID-19 outbreak, an isolation period, a period of extreme mental clarity, will do justice.

The goal is to build on your existing knowledge, give you the levers and capacity to do things on your own, not the instant fixes (there aren't any). Seeking help from an external source for something that is so deep rooted in the human system doesn't make sense, what you will read will make you internalise a few things. You had to someday, and it's my promise to make you do it by the end of your read.

I am free from this "fitness ferret wheel", at a ripe age of 22. This lets me pursue other forms of freedom. I sincerely hope that this book helps you attain that freedom in your own way, in your own life. If it has done that, in any amount, I'd be elated, for you.

INTRODUCTION

The idea of this book or what I thought for a while was a piece of "helpful written material that dovetails into ThBigFatFit's presence online" was 3 years in the running. Every moment (I exaggerate), of these 3 plus years I spent being obsessed about working out, eating right, cooking healthy, experimenting with diets, doing about every single thing that the "health and wellness" or the "fitness and food industry", in general, had to offer. Why? You ask? In these 3 years, I had gone through a riveting life-changing weight loss journey, an overall body transformation if you will. I had lost a total of 51 kilos. Yes, you read that right. If you haven't yet watched some of my YouTube videos or know about the channel. I make real life content on all things dieting/fitness, self care and what not. Let me take you back in time a little bit. I spent most of my childhood as an obese and close to morbidly overweight kid. I lived, breathed, walked, talked about food and eating, I still do, to an extent, but in a very, very different way, which you will soon figure out. At my peak, a 17 year old me, weighed 121 kgs/261 lbs. At the end of my first "cut", the weighing scale measured 69 kilos/152lbs, my leanest, a scrawny body with a six pack, a six pack with a layer of loose and saggy skin on top morphing the clarity anybody else at my body fat percentage would have. Don't worry, you will soon understand and comprehend all the buzzwords and fit jargon that you come across in this book, in fact it's important that you do. I will help you build up the groundwork. I still can't identify with my old self, not a single habit that I had back then resonates with me. I literally made 2 of me into one, close to half my body weight, gone, vanished.

I did this whole "feat" which I, my friends and family were proud of but not many of them know that 99% of the work was done in just under 12 months, with very little "super hard work". Yes. I do not want to discredit anybody who successfully loses weight but, it is a slippery slope with a proven process and for those who catch on to it, it has a great success rate. Everybody can do it. It may sound edgy, but "It ain't that hard". Yes I said it. Screw the motivation folks who obscure things and try to make it sound like it is. Do not worry, this book is not about my weight loss journey and the sob story behind it, nor is it a personal fat to fit memoir. It is also not a motivational screenplay. In fact, that sort of motivation wanes off. Thousands of people by hook or by crook lose weight, gain weight, some more than me, some less, props to all of them. Now there is an entire "weight loss" industry catering to millions of folks, but how I did it was awfully easy and it did not require a lot of help from the "fitness community" (or help from anybody). Just an 18-year-old curious mind was what it took.

This book is about a broader topic of learnings, demystification of concepts that are murky, tips that you would never know, tactics that are hidden from you, tricks that you can have up your sleeve when it comes to training, eating, exercising, dieting, call it whatever and living without having to sacrifice a SINGLE THING. YES, a single thing. (other than some time, energy and hard work, which I assumed was a given). The goal is to give the power to you. Make you live better through learning from the mistakes I and many like me made and continue to make. Give you a 3 year head start.

Have you ever wondered how your famous celeb folks can party, drink and eat all the junk but still when time comes, he or she gets in shape? Have you ever wondered if they gain or lose weight at all? Have you been astonished how some actors transform their body composition for every movie? Same goes with bodybuilders, MMA fighters, boxers and the like. They can magically go from fat or bulky to paper-thin shredded and aesthetic when time comes knocking. Well by the end of this read, you will soak in, grasp and build on those foundations, you can drink what you want (alcohol included), eat whatever you want, maintain a lifestyle of choice (as long as you are human) and look like your dream self. Yes, dream self.

So irrespective of whether you are thin, fat, obese, "skinny fat", tall, short or whatever, this book and what you will read will catapult you into a world of superpowers. Yes superpowers, as it will make you question the human species in general, their eating habits, dietary habits, activity habits. It'll make you appreciate the things that you never knew were so important. You will start questioning almost every ordinary thing that you do, that others do, you will implement new things in your life and if you follow the techniques and policies that are presented, in no time will you mimic behaviours of a "fitness trainer" or a "dietician" (did I mention I dissuade people from going to them other than outlier reasons? More on that later).

All this without an ounce of a headache to choose your workouts or diets or all the frustration that comes along with it. Just the contents of what you are about to read. Let me get you up to speed, we will be covering topics ranging from simple things like why humans eat in the first place, to what makes us move, to calorie counting, to FAD diets, to how your body reacts to HIIT (High intensity interval training) in a fasted state to how ketones can be your best friend. Well, did that last bit put you off? To clarify, this is not a science textbook, the subtitle of the book remains our main objective. Yes, we will touch just about every inch of the spectrum, but keep ourselves laser-focused on 1 thing, getting equipped to make better eating and fitness related decisions on a daily basis. The point of this book is not to clutter your mind with the jargonish info. All these topics are chosen because they form the BASE to HEALTH and WELLNESS in general.

It Is Deep Rooted in Society

You must have come across this fitness freak in your social circle. The guy or the girl who always wants to boast about what diet she is on. The one person who just lectures you (or anybody frankly) about food and dietary choices given the opportunity. The person who gloats about his current vegan-gluten free-ayurvedic-keto diet he or she is on (it's made up of course). This kind are many in society and I partly blame them for discouraging people and creating a negative impact on general health and fitness. Can you recall this person in your social group? Believe me, I was such a person, until I was socially feedbacked into thinking and doing otherwise, i.e, taking a chill pill. A guy who doesn't care about this aspect of life will get put off. It's like speaking about your favourite movie to a person who hasn't watched it. But these "gloaters" come from the right place, however. How can one help change other people and get them to look hotter, slimmer, thinner, fitter and eating right? There is no harm in doing this right? This could be your friend, better half, someone you date, parents, or even yourself. We will discuss this in length but everyone has this in this gene and it's hidden and sometimes it is in our subconscious. How much ever they might deny it. Everyone wants to be attractive, look their best and wants to do the diet, but the rampancy of misinformation, clutter and noise in the space precludes people from taking action. So will I provide you with the right information? No. That, you in your private life will gather. I will walk you through what we all forget to lay importance on, the fundamentals. De- noising is a very valuable talent when it comes to fitness. As much as it would pain the average joe to hear someone talk about fitness and gloating, by the end of this read you will know more than this average joe and be equipped to teach others, or not teach others and be selfish, which is okay and one can understand. Again, I would like to make it clear that I have taken a fundamentalist approach. Taking for granted that you will gain curiosity and build on this book. We will touch upon and strengthen the basics in a way like no other, these are the pillars of this part of life which is not life itself and we will not dig deep into some topics as they don't require us to".

We were born to live a life full of food and fun, evolutionarily, we as humans have progressed and lived a certain way, and that way is not keto or vegan or gluten-free or you following a diet.

That is my sincere belief. Sure, if you don't pay heed to things such as weight, health, wellbeing and fall back and hinder your body, you will have to take appropriate corrective measures and steps. But for that, it doesn't mean you have to become a fitness freak or a maniac. This thing is too simple for you to be getting a PhD as a normal human being whose life is not this. I see and know tons of people spending money, energy, resources, getting a personal trainer, a dietician, "online coaches", picking up stupid advice when their situation simply doesn't warrant it. Do not get me wrong, they are noble professions, but their requirement in this hi-tech world of information overload is very little. My analogy is this; would you go to a Neurosurgeon if you had a mild headache? Sure, chances of it being a tumour are undeniable, but what are the odds?

Taking a parallel, one (and I might get hate for this, but it is the reason I am writing this book for anyways) need not go to any dietician (it is almost a defunct career right now given so many diets come and go), or any form of fitness trainer for a weight loss, fat loss, weight gain, become fit or look better sort of a goal. There are obvious outliers to this, but the fact of the matter, for the majority remains. One has to channelise the little energy that they get towards the right thing rather than wasting it on superfluous wrong things. This energy, especially in fitness, is hard to find. If not made use of, it slips away.

Before You Read the Book:

I also want to set you up with some things in this introduction. I have been edgy, non conforming, controversial, blatant and unforgivingly honest throughout this book. This is because I am a science believing person, and every point that I make in this literature is fact based, research-based and this is dozens of months of research (that I did, mostly for myself). Sometimes, digging down papers, publishers, articles, podcasts, interviews and even old blog posts of experts in the field just so that I could make the point and make life easy for you. Even when you come across an opinion, be assured that it will be an experiential one (don't forget how I lost all that weight). We all have pre-existing biases, confirmation biases, and everything else that makes us boost our own ego. What mainly aids eliminate bias in this book is the fact that I do not proclaim or profess any single form of diet or type of exercise. I strictly oppose you from taking advice from a person who looks at life unidimensionally (at least their fitness life). This is exactly the reason I thought the idea of writing this book was a no brainer, it would help millions if not billions of people.

My Reasons for Writing This Book:

One of my core reasons for writing this book, and you can call it the largest reason, is to change the way people look at fitness, self care and food. You might think that it is a broad claim which it is, but I can clearly see the value, it is almost as if there is this secret pathway to reach enlightenment in this topic, the access to which the general population is denied. I say this as an industry insider. The industry in itself fragmented (not necessary for it to be at all) and is almost like a scheme, jumping from one fad to the other. I am an active member in this society. I work in the F&B (food and beverage) space and I am a "fitness geek" in my circles. Trust me when I say that the groundwork that you will be set up with, the revelations that you will have from this piece of literature will 100% change the way you look at fitness and food, you will be able to crack open gurus like an egg. That is a promise. Along with this, I was just tired of answering the same questions to everyone who knew my story. I needed a creative outlet parallel to usual work and business, writing was one. I couldn't hold back anymore with the misinformation, new fads propping up daily, people losing time, effort and money while I sat back and witnessed. That just did not sit well with me given that I have this potential and power to convey this in a very efficient manner through media.

With genuine skin in the game, given that I work in a related industry for a living, given I have a following for my content surrounding this, given that I have overseen close to 100+ life-changing transformations of people just by engaging with "TheBigFatFit" content with no personal trainer or fitness professional involved (yes, you don't need them) and my genuine need to be productive outside of daily work, writing what could be the most easily consumable piece of literature on this topic was worth taking a shot on. It would be dumb of me not to do this, almost a disservice I would say, you will soon realise why.

Don't get me wrong I am selfish, I wanted to work on myself before writing anything for others, but I did think by writing a piece of literature, I could use this vain thought to help others at the same time. Two birds one stone. You know a book puts your name out there and I am honest in agreeing with this vanity goal. This literature, however, could have been through a video, an article or a blog post, but no, I wanted to get it done with forever, help people live their best lives eating and training like "normal" human beings and still be able to look amazing, lose or gain weight, transform themselves into their dream person.

And for that, nothing better than a book. Not a small E-Booklet or a handbook of sorts (seriously) but an actual book that takes tremendous energy and patience to write and something you can read whenever, wherever (I suggest you read it how many ever times until things get etched in your brain and becomes second nature) and BOOM you're up to pace and you develop a layer of new knowledge in a new field or learnt about a new perspective and it will pay you back till you die.

The 4 Heroes of the Story:

On a concluding note of this introduction, I would like for you to carefully remember these 4 characters in my life, this is because I will allude to them throughout this book and they will help you cross reference and act as units of difference. Their main purpose is to help you grasp better and draw parallels and nothing else. Slowly, you will realise that many versions of these 4 characters exist in the real world. Many of them your friends, family, acquaintances and the like.

They are:

Kiara: 21, Height: 5ft 6 Inches, Weight: 53 kg

Open-minded, was plumpy in her childhood. Now has gotten into shape and has a decent idea about fitness and its concepts. She has tried multiple diets, this "low carb" thing her gym trainer told about worked best for her but she is still figuring out how to do something sustainable. Keeps gaining a layer of tummy when she slacks off and keeps working harder each time to get back to her best. Fitness for her = ferret wheel. Just started work at a Marketing Agency.

Aunt Ruchi: 38, Height: 5ft 2 inches, Weight: 75 kg

Punjabi, loves to eat and cook. Was athletic, fit and slim in her early and tender years, but now has put on more weight than she can handle. Joint pains, breathlessness and stress eating greasy, tasty North Indian junk is a habit. Wonders what went wrong most of the time. She could do with being able to move around freely. Homemaker. (Husband is a restaurateur FYI. owns 3 restaurants)

Michael: 29, Height 6ft 1 Inch, Weight: 82 kg. Body Fat: 9% Muscle Mass: 69 kg

Eccentric, ate meat, took supplements, gear (commonly known steroids, anabolics, roids, juice) and lifted hardcore weights for 10+ years. With a rekindled love for animals, he has now gone vegan. Works out Crossfit style 6 x a week, does extra cardio on the rest day. "Preps" his meals for the week every Sunday night. Spends more on his food/body than any other single line item on his personal financial statement. Investment Banker. Phew!

My Dad: 54, Height: 5ft 8inches, Weight: 77

No weight or major health problems, was skinny and fairly athletic in his early years, metabolism is god's best gift to him. He has slowly but surely gotten bigger in size over the years. Does little to no exercise. Life is good, really doesn't give a damn about weight, fitness or anything surrounding it. Does go for the occasional walk. Makes fun of his beloved son. Will not miss his scotch for anything though. Mechanical Engineer.

CHAPTER 1

WHY DO WE EAT?

Starting from scratch, questioning the very basics.

Scene: On a day when I was out with Michael and the boys to play football.

Right after the intense 60 min game, everyone was dehydrated. As they should be. There is a golgappa wala right outside the rent and play arena. 2 folks went straight for it, while still gasping for breath from the feisty game they just played. 3 more folks went to the adjacent shop to buy a soft drink, 2 sipped red bull from the branded vending machine. I and Michael, looking at each other, baffled, sipping on water with just one more friend of ours. 3 out of 12 were interested in water.

I looked at him and said "What a weird world we live in". For us food meant something and for others something else. "Bro, you should this new age sprinting technique..." Michael rambled on.

Ask yourself; What kind of a person are you?

Do you eat because you have to? Do you eat because you love to? Do you always eat? Do you almost never eat? Are you a foodie? Are you carefully planning your meals so that it fits in your diet and body goals? Or are you a, "Don't care, just feed me when I am hungry" kind of a person?

You see, throughout history, the present we live in and probably for the considerable future, we have learned, are learning and will learn that we eat because we are hungry. That's what most of our minds have been conditioned to hear as the explanation. Hunger is such an uncomfortable feeling, right? Just thinking about it feels annoying. It is not a pleasant thing. If you analyse this at a deeper level, you get to know that our body needs energy, and food gives us that energy. What a simple and tactful explanation It is exactly right that food gives us energy, nothing new in that. Factually it is the primary energy source and the major contributor for where we get the energy to be able to function, we as humans cannot possibly think of altering our chemical and biological selves to take anything else to fuel us. If we were phones, that is our battery %, it need not always be at a 100% or at extremely low levels, these are not optimal, but we need it to survive. Why am I giving you this primary schoolboy explanation? Well for starters, we as a 21st-century population have BLATANTLY forgotten about it. Food is energy? No, this does not strike us as such. I mean really, ask yourself. When is the last time you said, "Hey I am out of energy, I need to eat something that brightens my mood and performance levels". Heck no, you were "starving" so you grabbed a snickers. Or it was lunch break and you just gulped food without reason throwing out the concept of hunger. There was a damn good chance you weren't hungry. Take it from me.

Food has now become a lifestyle, a hobby, a profession, a way of expression, an obsession, a business for some, a blessing for the poverty-stricken and an overflowing commodity for the well off. Somewhere between its invention, the stone ages, the middle ages, and the present, we have lost track of what food is to us. To draw a parallel, food is so paramount and vital to us that it determines how much we weigh, how we look, how our body feels, how our body functions, and so many critical things which you will learn of soon. A major section of the current population does not and will not ever get this. Please, as a reader of this book and for your own benefit I ask of you to open your eyes to see what food is actually making you do. Ask how it makes you feel. What is your relationship with food like? What happens to your body on its consumption and also in its absence. Yes, both. Although for some like aunt Ruchi, there is no concept of absence of food. It's in the system, always. Such people will never learn.

Mark my words, etch them in your mind, but what you are about to read should be drilled into your subconscious. How I have postulated it is - food or every consumption has 3 types of effects. Short, Medium and Long term.

Short Term Effects:

Does your stomach grumble in hunger? - Food

Do you feel a bit happy after sipping that coke? - Food

Do you feel sleepy after a wholesome meal? - Food

Do you feel regretful after that bad-tasting lunch? - Food

Do you feel dizzy all of a sudden on an empty stomach? - Food

Do you feel a bit crappy after that greasy meal? - Food

Do you feel tipsy and adventurous after a couple of drinks? - Food

For Medium-Term Effects, Food Determines;

How you look.

How your body composition is (beer belly or flat stomach)

How much you weigh.

How your internal organs have taken to it.

How easily you move around.

For Long Term Effects, Food Determines;

Your overall health,

Your immunity,

Your bodily functions,

Your diseases and so many other things.

Food for your body is energy, yes, but DATA more.

You see how goddamn important food is, have you looked at it ever this way? You see you can't just eat for the sake of eating (one side of the spectrum). Or eat whatever and whenever (the other side of the spectrum). If you do either, you are doomed. You will find yourself blaming society, past events, lack of exercise, your family, your genetics or a million other reasons as justifications for how you look and feel whenever you worry about your body all of a sudden.

I don't think it's just me who on a random Wednesday afternoon, suddenly gets body conscious after looking in the mirror. It just hits me out of nowhere. Crying over spilt milk. I was in this very position when I weighed 121 kilos walking around like a mini elephant. But the journey that got me to the 70s and I am a fit man mind you, with a solid body (all year) and how I think about this daily commodity of food is what got me to help other people think of it differently. My god what a superpower it was, just by altering my mind and very little real energy put towards learning the science behind consumption, macronutrients/micronutrients, dietary habits, their effects on the human body, (more in detail on this in the future) and in essence looking after what goes into my mouth during this riveting weight loss journey, I was able to not only control how I look feel on a short/medium term basis, I could also sense if somebody else was doomed. I could sense people in my social circle that would "mysteriously gain weight" like Kiara did so often or "got that beer belly" or their health took a bad turn or even cases where their overall body composition started deteriorating. I even warned some of them looking at their habits, they did not listen. You see that is why these "fit nerds" keep giving you unsolicited advice. Michael would advise you about this till your ears dropped off.

Before you think, "Hey, I have never been fat or unfit, I am thin (fairly okay) and not a gym freak. I always manage to stay thin and there is no chance I need to change things. I will die like this", wait till I burst your happy bubble soon. You are also doomed. But in about 5-10-15 years depending on how many lucky stars you are carrying. These people are or end up being "skinny fat"- skinny fat means you appear skinny from far but have fat stored in common areas giving you a very unstructured and un--aesthetic look. Like a layer of love handles or saggy chest. You are thin but not toned either. My dad falls in this category.

Once we forget the basics of what food's job in this world is, we tend to forget that it is so powerful, I reiterate, there are very few energy sources other than that our body knows, it's our fuel. I massively benefitted from looking at it this way. And if the fuel is messed up, or is present in too little or too much quantity, there will be massive ramifications that the overall vehicle has to face.

So in essence, I want you guys, not to become food scientists or food nerds, but to please look at food for what it actually is rather than just something that gives momentary pleasure or satisfies the taste buds. Not just as delicious dishes but as actual energy that you require, not too much, not too little, just the right amount and your body will signal you when to start and stop consuming. Therein lies the secret to freedom.

This mindset is the first block of cement in our goal to be able to achieve Nutritional Freedom, i.e, eat whatever you want and still jog on with a six-pack or stay lean or stay your optimal best.

SO YES, PLEASE UNDERSTAND WHY YOU EAT?

Exercise: What Goes in My Mouth, Goes in the Book!

Write down what you eat for 1 week.

Just for 1 week, start from a Monday, just make a note, on your phone or on paper, what you exactly ate.

This includes all meals snacks, water even. Whatever particular thing you eat or drink, goes written or typed.

Time duration of one week is compulsory. Don't try to be presumptuous, don't cheat or eat healthy just because you are doing this. Be you, but note it down somewhere.

At the End:

I want you to have a clear list of what you consumed, Monday to Sunday.

Total number and names of distinct meals and dishes.

Times at which you ate.

It should result in a very simple note.

This will come of use later as you go on reading.

CHAPTER 2
WHAT DO WE EAT?

Cognisance of what exactly goes in your pie-hole. A lot more than just pies.

Scene: *Kiara and me in uni during lunch hour*

Kiara – "What is this chicken and egg salad you eat for lunch everyday? Doesn't it bore you? They say too much meat is bad for digestion. Shouldn't you eat some fruits too? Isn't that what experts say?

Me – "I am going to dumb this down as much as possible because that is how I learnt it, that is how the most effortlessly fit people know it and I believe, that is how anybody would ever get interested to learn it, else, these "fitness experts" and people in the field will make this sound like a nuclear project and push people away from a chance at a wonderful, fit and tasteful life" paraphrasing what I said before I had the first fitness talk during Lunch hour with Kiara.

We are surrounded by food, think about it, an average person has at least 3 meals a day, which you will soon realise is way too much, this means, per week it amounts to 21, per month it is at least 600 meals, that's at least 7200 times you eat in a year, WOW. That's A LOT. A lot for 365 days. Our bodies were not designed to eat that much. Well, we could eat any quantity but definitely not at that frequency. We need to realise this now. Adding to this, these are all not the same meals, this habit has diversity and variance, different cuisines, servings, serving sizes, snacks, beverages. Adding to that, events, festivals, parties etc mean that the 7200 times that you are consuming meals are a conservative figure. They say an average person should minimise trivial decision making and keep the brain ready for important and critical decisions, well 7200 decisions on something as rudimentary as food are being made every year. For some folks like Aunt Ruchi, this is the most important decision she would be making for the day.

Now, why did I bring this point up?;

I tell this because we are going to take the same decision making capacity and use it towards something else, something that does not eat into your bandwidth, something that can be ingrained in your subconscious and in turn, helps you maintain shape and help you achieve nutritional freedom.

It was a realization to us that for us to look and feel a certain way, you need to master and take control of food (yes food first, we will get to exercise). Well to be able to have some control, you need to watch what you eat and what you don't. And to be able to do that, you need to know what exactly is food? I mean scientifically, what does food consist of? Please ask yourself this schoolboy question - What is in food? No really, what is inside it? Write down your answers.

If your answers are something on the lines of bread, veggies, corn, chicken, you're not wrong, but you're way off. At that stage, they still remain food by definition, if that wasn't what you thought of, what exactly did you think of? I want you to question it this way; What is in that bread? What is in that chicken? What is in that vegetable?

The Idea of FQ, Just like IQ and EQ

Did you think of something else when answering the last paragraph? This really shows your food FQ (Food Quotient). I believe in this post obesity epidemic world, FQ should be a high priority given that we think about it more than money, art and science which are usually taught in schools.

Well if we keep going down this thought lane of "what really is in food", we figure out that they are like all things on the universe, made of some atoms and molecules (matter). But the gold mine is found when we just take a couple of steps back. Our scientists have named them macronutrients and micronutrients. There, these are what majorly constitute food. Not a discovery, but still very integral. For the purposes of this book, let us not deviate to more than macronutrients, micronutrients and fibre (the 3rd somewhat major) component. (Water and other negligible components also exist but we aren't doing a science lecture here, far from it). What you learned in the previous chapter is a perfect stack for us to build on. I believe in taking a step by step approach, the thought experiments that you encountered in the last chapter should have set you up enough to go down the road which I believe will help you own eating habits and living life to the fullest. Food is one of man's greatest inventions and as we continue to innovate in this field, make tasty, exciting and resourceful new foods, trust me we do not need to live a miserable life of abstinence.

"The World of Macros and Micros"

"Macros" as the fitness and wellness community calls it has probably single handedly changed and made lives. Macros are short for macronutrients, these are **Protein, Fats and Carbs. PCF or macros in short**, you learnt about this in 4th grade and forgot about it. I can probably call this the most important word used in this book.

"Micros", short for micronutrients, on the other hand, are the important vitamins and minerals. Again, components essential for your survival and functioning of the body. That's it, this is what food is made of, that is what gives you energy and these 2 in combination are the base to every single food or drink that is ever made out there in the world.

The day that I learned that each food particle has a different composition (split) of these macros and micros was a game-changer. I was probably at the gym researching about dieting in between sets while this happened. Better yet, uncovering that each and every macro or micro has an effect on your body and how the body reacts to them is different is still fresh in my memory. (We shall elaborate more on this later). I remember having a lesser serving of rice that day. You will figure out just why.

If I can make it sound practical, having a sandwich for lunch instead of having a steak makes a world of a difference. Having paneer/tofu instead having potatoes is a huge difference. Having eggs vs having pancakes for breakfast is not even an apples to oranges comparison, it's even wide apart. They are not just "lunch/breakfast/dinner options" anymore.

Look at food as energy and the fact that this energy, as a concept can be broken down into two; Macros and Micros. What we are going to talk about next is the dreaded most disdainful word in the so-called "fitness industry". The term "CALORIE". A demon for most, a friend for many. Calories are a double-edged sword. If you know it well enough you will be thankful. If you know it because it exists, you will always look at it with disdain. I posit that however basic the term, the importance is always understated.

My dad despises this word with all his heart. Michael just has to say this word 5 times a day otherwise he is not satisfied.

The time has come for me to drill one more core concept to boost your FQ. The calorie is the representation of the energy we get from food. The calorie is nothing, and nothing but nomenclature for this "food energy". When I told you food consists of PCF, did you ever think of how this was calculated or measured? How was this quantified? I wouldn't want to give you a dictionary explanation. That would defeat the purpose and as a curious person who picked up this book, I expect you to be your 21st century self to research about every single point of topic and build on your knowledge. Some might do it, some won't. So here goes.

The next part is something that calls upon the left side of the brain, wash and clean your cognitive, analytic and mathematical mind as you head towards reading it. I am going to put it out in as simple a way as possible without making it sound jargonish.

The SI unit of energy is called the Joule, (SI Unit - Measuring standard, universally accepted), colloquially, kilojoule (joule x 1000) is what was used to measure energy from food, now it is the calorie (1 calorie = 4.2 kJ). Screw the math, all you need to know is food consists of calories, which you already did know, but now you know what calories mean and what are in those calories. **Hint:** PCF. (Plus fibre mostly) As we live in a world where hardly people measure food in kJ (but if they do, you know how to convert them to calories), and as you must know, calories have taken the world by storm, we will stick to talking about calories or kcal (both are same) as you might see them expressed in many cases. THAT'S IT, IF YOU HAVE A DEEP UNDERSTANDING OF THE CALORIE (or kcal) + Macros + Micros, you have won half the battle.

The Holy Macro Math

A thing that people overlook is the fact that PCF are all different. It's not just food, it's not just calories, it's not taste and size but they are different by name, different by nature, different in occurrence and different in the way they work. These little things have huge ramifications short, medium and long term biologically. Having this in mind, it is time to uncover another hidden gem that circles almost your entire life. Counting calories. You'd think why on earth you'd want to do that. Remember, mini sacrifices, huge pay offs. Before we reach mastery levels and learn how to count the calories in anything that you eat without any help, let us take the first step in this endeavour, the ability to read and understand the nutritional labels at the back of your packaged goods.

The math is this, and this will help you read all nutritional labels. Anything ever printed.

1 gram of protein = 4 calories

1 gram of carbohydrate = 4 calories

1 gram of fat = 9 calories.

And, 1000 grams or 1 kg of actual weight = 7,700 calories (do not forget this). If you gained a kilo or lost a kilo, this is where it came from.

Each gram of the said macro has the said amount of calories (PCF = 449, remember it this way). This last sentence would get my dad to sleep, but you will soon realise that if he took the time to read the book (which I know he will), life would be different.

Common Food Sources: Macro Wise Illustration

*this is a map, not the territory.

I have laid this out for context reasons and not as a table of information. The more you build on this in real life, the more will be adept at knowing this. This is not a cookbook. But, for the most part, and the majority of the population, this brief, in itself will go a long enough way. All of the PCF occurs naturally, but, some are also processed (don't read this as bad, because that is not the insinuation). There are so many more food sources than what you are about to read but I look at it at this way, either its natural or it is man made, man enhanced. That gives us 2 buckets to put food sources rich in each and every one of the PCF. Beyond this, all knowledge on this topic (for me as well as I continue to learn new things) is welcome.

Protein Rich Sources:

We have **processed** protein in Whey, Soy/Plant-based protein powders. Then, we have **natural** dried versions, lean versions, different cuts of meat in Chicken, Veal, Beef, Pork, Egg Whites. Then we have Milk-based items in Cheese, Tofu, Paneer and Plant-based items in Legumes, sprouts etc.

Carbohydrate Rich Sources:

We have **processed** carbs in – Cola, Syrups, Sweeteners, Jams and Mass produced baked goods. We have **natural** Sugars or Simple Carbs in fruits, juices, table sugar itself, honey etc. Then we have starch or complex carbs in rice, bread, cooked grains, pasta, corn, etc

Fat Rich Sources:

We have **natural** oils, nuts, egg yolks, etc. Fats are also present in red meat and fish in a greater concentration. We also have **processed** cheese, butter, fried items, packaged and baked goods.

*Processed here means that the food undergoes some sort of factory synthesis.

Case in Point: PCF are Not Mutually Exclusive.

Protein high foods, don't just have protein, same goes for carbohydrate and fat high foods. That is why I used the word "rich" in all three of the last 3 sub headings. The concentration of the said macro is higher but by and large, they have all of PCF in them in some or the other proportion. And also, food, as a farm produce, is not the same around the world which means quality and quantity changes as we move across geographies.

So, mixtures exist. Some foods are protein + fat heavy = cheese, some foods are fat and carb-heavy = doughnut. It is paramount to take them for what it is, there is no rocket science here.

Now the type of carbohydrate (like sugar or starch), type of protein (type of amino acids), type of fats (saturated, unsaturated, etc) is immaterial here, that is Michael talk, in fact, within those types, there are multiple subcategories and so on and so forth which is again, important for science but tangential to our objective. So forgive me if you were waiting for the "tell me more about carbs explanation". I will reiterate again that I have taken a fundamentalist approach to looking at food, I will not posit a theory nor represent half-truths just because I need to convince a certain section of the society. The goal should be to improve your food IQ or FQ as I call it, much beyond your reading of this book. It pays you back in heaps.

Your macros are named differently because they have different functions and they behave differently. I have relied on the concept of absorption in my mind to understand this better and in fact easier, absorption or use of the PCF by your body is what people call metabolism. It is a chemical process. It happens at a cell level. A very, very key concept in achieving your fitness and nutritional freedom.

Carbs are absorbed or metabolised the quickest, easy to digest and energy is transferred to the body rapidly.

They are immediately converted into what you will learn to be very important - glucose. Some carbs digest more quickly than the other. In the order of digestibility sugar (simple carbs) > starch (complex carbs).

The Michael's of the world would throw in a harangue about Glycemic Index, but, we aren't fighting for our food PhDs right now.

Proteins are absorbed the second-fastest.

Fats are absorbed last, this is often used by our body as a reserve (4th-grade deja vu again) and;

Fibre, a type of carbohydrate is not "digestible" by the human body. However, it's importance is so much that it is regarded often as an extension to the PCF, although it is part of the C to begin with.

Anything you garner in your private life about these is welcome knowledge but beyond the scope of this book. I wish to stay focused and convey this in a manner that helps you obviate daily food and fitness problems.

The World of Packaged Foods (No They Are Not Bad)

I would here ask of you another favour. A favour that you would do for yourself on behalf of me. Go to the nearest packaged food (raw or finished) that you can find and try deciphering what is written in the back (at least the macros) for now. Do it now. In fact get 2 or 3 items before you read the next few sentences. Trust me, this will help. If you do not have anything lying around which definitely should not be the case, get your phone and google the image of the nutritional label of any packaged food of your choice, again raw or finished. Raw as in meat or flour, finished as in a chocolate bar or ice cream.

Read the protein, read the carbohydrate, read the fat content. Then, read the whole serving size. Are the details given for the serving size or are they given for the whole package? Have they even mentioned the serving size? Just reading the label is never enough as the data might just be for one serving while you may think that the entire pack is worth that many calories as what the label is suggesting. Serving sizes are very important, always and always check the serving size and the total net weight of the pack. Serving sizes may also be in the form of "per 50g" or "per 100g" kind of representation. Nevertheless, always look out for them before doing the calculation.

A small example here goes a long way, an ice cream tub might read 236 calories in big font on the front of the package. But at the back, you see 236 calories per serving size of 30 grams. (they carefully mention the serving size elsewhere in the package or morph it). Some also dupe people by claiming that it is 236 calories per scoop. Now how much is a scoop actually? Scoops differ in sizes. You will have to search around to realize that it is 236 calories per scoop which is 30 grams and that it has 10 servings which means it is a 300 gram pack and that it amounts to 2360 calories. That is how the average joe (Aunt Ruchi) gets played. That is a lot and it is dense. Do not worry, the regulatory bodies in food have now made sure that in some or the other way, all information is presented. That is what obesity did to us.

This is just an example, one of the easiest actually, but you will have to read, reread the preceding paragraphs, again and again, to register it in your mind. Why I hint on this is because there are millions of such packaged foods in production and some are more complicated to read and one can get a hold of this only by experience. Once you have this skill, you will be able to tell how many calories (with macros) your favourite dish at your favourite restaurant has. Without even flinching. Well, you will be close, not exact but that is damn well amazing as that is all you need. Kiara is close, she can almost at this point approximate the calories of any dish, but she is still learning, practising and researching. We will dig deeper into this topic when the time comes.

You will make more use of the holy macro math and take great benefits of its use in the future chapters but try to memorise this, more so, internalise this. This will only help you and make wiser day to day decisions. Knowing what you eat is a superpower, once you know this, you can gain weight at will, lose weight at will, eat whatever you want, drink whatever you like, feel like a boss because you know exactly what went in your body, and how your body is going to absorb it. Just wait till you know what you can do with this power and where you can use it (I make the evil laugh) SO YES, PLEASE UNDERSTAND WHAT YOU EAT!

EXERCISE: Reading the Right Tables!

For the next 30 days, every package food, raw or finished, will have its backside nutritional label read by you.

You will read not only its nutritional label, but figure out the total calories, split up of all macros and frankly every little piece of information that you can find. Sugar, fibre, tom, dick, harry, expressed in whatever quantity, whatever way, please turn to the label, read like you would the news.

I want you to understand, read everything right from the licenses, trademarks, making process to ingredients to whether it is gluten-free or non-GMO or vegan or anything for that matter that they claim.

Research more about whatever new terms you come across and also dig into the "claims" they make. You have to follow this for 30 days.

Make a reminder on your phone, that helps you remember every morning that packed foods should be read, thoroughly.

CHAPTER 3

WHY DO PEOPLE MOVE?

No really, why do people indulge in activities beyond what their normal lives require them to, are they mad?

Scene: Me and my Dad on a normal day

My dad: "The coronavirus has forced all gyms to shut, Will you become fat again?"

Me: "Haha, It doesn't work like that dad. Period.

Dad: So you will not gain weight because you left the gym?

Me: "What if I had a life threatening injury and can never visit the gym? If I just exercised my way to being where I am, I am doomed. "What if I moved to antarctica taking my diet out for a toss? If I just dieted my way to being where I am. I am doomed"

Me speaking with my dad on the stupidity of people who just do 50% of the work. If we look at our body's fitness as a government policy. Please regulate food, but also regulate exercise. We need to do both.

Start from Your Social Circle:

Do you know that fit uncle, fit aunt or a fit older family friend or an acquaintance that maintains their body and looks younger than his or her age? Genetics aside, you can make out that this took some sort of effort from their side. Does that remind you of somebody? If not think of one such person right now, every social circle has one at least, I had many.

Back in the day, as a curious person who was fascinated about this topic, I went up to these folks when I had the chance and asked them a few questions. This was a general conversation topic for me. (And this is a general conversation topic for anybody interviewing Anil Kapoor)

After the cliched "Hey/how are you doing/what's going on, etc" I jumped to;

What is the secret to your good looks at this age?" or "What is the secret to your good shape?" or "How do you manage to look like that?"

I made a few inferences from a series of such interactions. Yes, off late I started to ask this or slide this topic into almost anybody who was in conversation with me. Fit, Fat or anywhere in between. Flattery really is a tool I tell you, it works.

Summarising My Inferences, I'd Say This:

Ask any such question to a fairly experienced man or a woman 40+ and they will say just 2 things, *"Right food and exercise, broadly"*

Now ask this to a person who is below 40-45 age range?

Even though they are not wrong, they will give you some advanced answers. Things like *"Drink lots of water, go for a jog daily or join the gym"* (or something in this cadre).

Now, ask this to someone who is below 30.

Here is where things get dangerous. Answers like *"Don't eat carbs after 6, lift light weights for more reps"*. Classic Michael.

On the flip side, if someone wasn't taking care of themselves, they would address the elephant in the room and say.

"I don't watch what I eat or exercise, you're being too nice"

Now if you ask me or any fit geek, you'd get advanced answers, but mainly, primarily, fundamentally, it revolves around diet and exercise or as we like to call it, nutrition and training, or if we take a few steps back, food and activity. BASIC THINGS. This is something you can do for yourself, asking people. Scanning the market. The answers will fall in the same context - food and activity. It is such a generic answer, right? No rocket science, just mundane things. How could we mess this up? I thought. But, broadly, people are not wrong, across the spectrum of age, skill level and experiences, they simplify and tell you that the key to staying fit revolves around those 2 things. It is not that simple if you look at folks like my aunt as examples but it is that simple in the fact that it revolves around these two. It was very transformative for me the day I identified and locked in this theory in my mind. You see there is nothing complex in there, while we demystified the former up until now (FQ), let's now delve into demystifying the latter, AQ (Activity Quotient).

Given that we cannot amass all the knowledge in the world about exercise, all we need to aim at is the right knowledge, knowledge and information that helps us, things that we almost ought to know, insights that are obfuscated by many in the field. And to begin this process, I thought I needed to take the same approach that we did for food, get back to history, understand basics and define it for what it is. We are not biochemists to research on food and its components to no end nor are we physiologists or kinesiologists (study of exercise and movement) to do the same for activity and exercise, these are professions, what we are looking for is real-world truths that are actionable, that is it. The simplicity of it all will benefit us and only that. We need something like > energy > food > calories >macros > micros > how and why they matter? But for exercise. Once you connect the dots, you can definitely up the skill and learn about tips and tricks. I have taken the same approach to exercise.

We will not be studying research articles about how much muscle mass in pounds Arnold Schwarzenegger (Bodybuilder, Actor, Politician) had and what exercise and how many repetitions and in what variations he did them that got him there but we would be touching upon 21st-century basics that will lead you to understand almost everything and aid practical usage. Remember, the aim is to be your own trainer.

That takes us way back to understanding the holy grail of activity. That is how I'd like to think of it, that for me, is the base to every single brick ever laid on the building of exercise.

Have you ever questioned why we move? Other than doing our daily activities, why do people exercise? Why do some people play sport? Why do some people move their body and play around with weights at the gym? Are they crazy? Why do people stretch before doing physical activity? Why do people do yoga? Why is certain people's posture always good? Why are some people more flexible?

Take note that not everybody has the same type of body. Not because God made us that way (which is true) but because some people work on their bodies. People are different across the board. They have different body shapes, length, breadth, height. Have you mindfully questioned why this is so ever? Have you observed how people's muscular structure, their overall look is not the same?

Think of the Weight of Your Body as a Mathematical Equation:

A - B = ± C, where A is How much you are eating (calories), B is how much you are burning (calories), and C is the value of the difference, which is your current body weight being added or subtracted on a daily basis. This is a very important equation, we will touch upon this multiple times from now and will form the basis of your understanding of a multitude of things.

We won't get to how this equation doesn't work for growing children and senior citizens as that is tangential to the topic. But, after you have stopped "growing naturally", i.e, your growth hormone takes the backseat, you are post puberty and are not growing any taller. This is pretty much the equation your body follows.

Write this down, copy it, save it somewhere, YOUR BODY IS THE SUM TOTAL OF HOW MUCH YOU ARE CONSUMING MINUS HOW MUCH YOU ARE BURNING OFF (USING FOR ENERGY). We are going to probe into the burning off part now. You see, we absorb this magical energy from food, this energy is dispensed for the normal functioning of the body and day to day movements and activity that we do. Now our movement can range from walking, talking, getting up, moving, sliding, falling, climbing, anything that involves movement and energy expenditure from the body. EACH AND EVERY ACTIVITY BURNS CALORIES or USES CALORIES (calories = energy). That is why you see these cringey quotes saying the body burns 10 calories when you smile and 5 calories when you to frown. (Those numbers are made up, but you get my point)

You see the body is constantly balancing energy, if you are consuming more than you are burning, you will gain weight, if you are burning more than you are consuming, you will lose weight. This is what the truth is. This fact is undefeatable. WOW! Right? That is why we get to the second of 2 pillars of this book, Activity or exercise. If you want to look a certain way, controlling and knowing about food helps but if you want to accentuate yourself, exercise (I'd like to call it training) will give you an edge.

That is why for years before we can remember, we have been doing activity, moving our bodies, playing sport, doing labour, doing functional things like daily chores. This is how yoga, martial arts, weight lifting and cardio vascular training that we see today originated. From as long as we can go back, exercise or movement was part of human civilisation. It evolved along with us. People who do more activity (exercise) burn off more energy, hence "having control" over their weight, there is no chance they just magically gain weight. They are just doing too much activity, burning more than an average joe. That is why Gordon Ramsay eats like an animal but is super slender. He just works out like crazy.

If they do gain weight, then the only justification is that one of the variables A or B has changed. Either A has increased or B has reduced. People who do no activity or lesser activity than general consumption will gain weight. And this is the exact narrative is why people recommend training or exercise for you to stay in shape. That is the patent importance of exercise, that is why we move and that is why we exercise from a blinkered, narrow point of view which is true and it does the job. But have you come across someone who says "I work out, I exercise and I still have not lost a single kilo" or "I am not seeing any results"?? Over the long run I have seen "do exercise or maintain diet" just doesn't cut it. You have to be willing to push through the pushbacks.

This is more like an aerial understanding of fitness. Our goal, however, is to get deeper for once, clean the bottom and never get back there again, just build on this trench. What I mean here is to unlearn things that you may have already learned. Our goal is also to know the vital differences between exercises and routines and see what fits our lifestyle and what works best for you, choosing and doing the form of exercise you love and grow to love. Something that does not bore you. This may be Yoga, Pilates, Weightlifting, Zumba or anything that you choose. You see as we learnt, fundamentally exercise is meant to "burn off energy". That is the big takeaway. Some people do it as a habit, some people as an obsession and some people as a compulsion. But we do it anyway. So yes, UNDERSTAND WHY WE MOVE/ DO ACTIVITY.

EXERCISE: A Day in the Life!

Whenever you get time,

I want you to wilfully spend one day with the most fittest person you know accompanying them in all their meals.

I want you to do the same thing with the fattest person you know (adjusted for age). Adjusted for age meaning, fat and young not fat because of age and health reasons.

Okay, if you cannot spend a whole day, try, at the very least, spending a few hours with 1 meal in the bare minimum with them.

I want you to carefully observe them in their natural habitat and try to discern as many things as possible, external and internal, behavioural and physical, all aspects.

No writing, no notes, be present, be observant. That is all I ask of you.

CHAPTER 4

WHAT DO PEOPLE CONSIDER EXERCISE TO BE?

An exhaustive approach to understanding what it does.

Scene: I was at Aunt Ruchi's place and this is what I over hear. A kitty party chat. I was probably 15 years old here. I am paraphrasing.

"My god you have put on weight, you should try Yoga."

"Walking is the best exercise",

"Running is the best for weight loss",

"Pilates is the best for toning your body" (whatever that means)

"Weightlifting is the best for becoming big and muscular"

"Crossfit is the best and most complete form of workout, I heard it on the internet"

"Power yoga can make you lose 3 kgs of "fat" in just one week" (haha)

This is how the common fitness war plays out. A debate about who and what is best. Very few deem it important to question this though, my dad would literally not bat an eye while my aunt would believe anyone. Kiara would be stuck in a whirlwind and you know Michael, he'd be running the debates. You see everyone needs and wants only results. Most don't care about the journey, they want to get to the destination, quick. So they need the so-called "quickest" path. I do not blame them. But, the world we live in today as compared to the 1900s or even early 2000s, has a ton of "workout options". With variety we also have a problem; The problem off "WHICH ONE DO I CHOOSE?", "WHICH ONE WILL GIVE ME RESULTS?" and the most dangerous "WHICH IS THE SHORTCUT?"

It's about Sustenance:

My sincere request is to you is to shift this mindset now, try asking yourself "WHICH ONE WORKS FOR MY GOALS (goals can range from I need to move my body often to I need to lose a 100 kilos) AND WHICH ONE DO I MOST LIKE DOING". Yes, most "like doing". These two questions will be a game changer when it comes to how you look at exercise. Because, this is not summer camp. It's something that you make a part of life.

Sustenance is the absolute key. This kind of thinking changed my life, my transformation and as I have witnessed, many others'. Kiara had a choice. Elongated period of success in terms of being in her most optimal (optimal not best) shape, OR, 2 months of rigorous work only to burn herself out and get back to where she was. The good old fitness ferret wheel. What would a wise person choose?

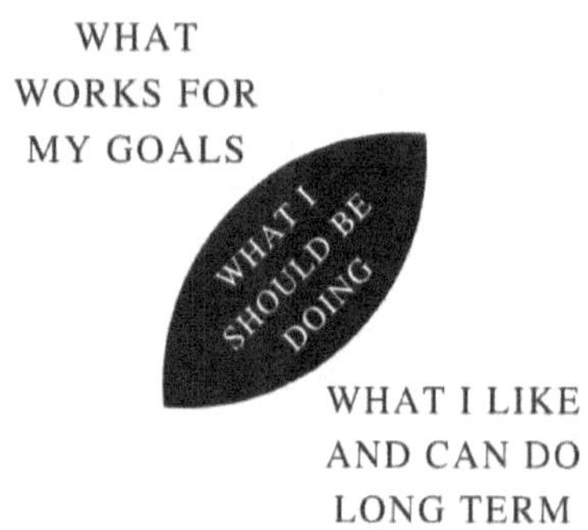

WHICH ONE WORKS FOR MY GOALS AND WHICH ONE DO I MOST LIKE DOING = WHICH ONE YOU SHOULD BE DOING

The 2 circles don't always match, but if you gain a clear understanding of pillars upon which the forms of exercise were built, you can mix/match and create your own routines and gain complete freedom. You see that was our plan from the start. You will make minute sacrifices but overall, you will not be a mentally fatigued person. If you have lost the mental battle, the physical self has no chance, it might sound cliched but it's the truth. Something that any person, who has miserably, forcibly, unsustainably and inauthentically lost weight or "made a body" clearly knows. People do it for movies, some for a "wedding", some for a "fashion show" and so on. For these folks, a relapse is waiting. Sooner or later, it is. I have faced it. Hundreds of thousands of people achieve these quick transformations in a very fastidious, strict and controlled manner. They create short term war zone environments that they will not be able to replicate lifelong. Sooner or later, you will take shape to represent your authentic self. You are bound to relapse, many "fit dudes" who got jacked following a "6 week workout plan" (same goes for diets). 2 or 3 years later are back where they started, a shadow of their self. It's like taking a crash course to "get it over with". Other than rare examples, they do tend to put on weight or "lose the abs" or "lose muscle" "lose strength" etc. Unsustainable, short term diets, workout plans, substance abuse to make a quick transformation will burn you out. With exercise, it is more so the case. You can boot camp your way out of a couple of kilos but your entire life cannot be a continuous Boot Camp. Again, build lifestyles, not diets and workout plans. Diets and Workout plans have their place but only to accentuate and "get you ready", not to dictate how you live.

An example here would be me and cardio. Thanks to tons of research, trial and error, I can get away with doing less of it. I can, Michael cannot. He is bound. Both have similar bodies. (Mine with lose skin however). I did minimal cardio but the right type of cardio during my journey. That is unheard of if anyone has ever lost more than 10 kilos. How? You will soon figure out. But for now understand that you will be able to get away with things, be abnormal, be challenging the status quo set by your "fit gurus" and still be able to achieve results, for that we need to set you up with the right arsenal of knowledge.

Even a kid knows exercise in general burns calories (energy) off, that is its primary *result* of exercise, but not necessarily its primary *function*. It is an outlet of energy, and this energy need not always come from food. What if you have not eaten at all today and you decide to work out? What will exercise do then? Exercise is a way in which we can use up the energy that we have, be it food or energy that we already stored in our body across places. It is by far the biggest tool other than food to manage the energy balance of the body which is the key indicator of how we look and how much we weigh. Given this fact, whichever form of exercise burns the most calories should be the best for weight loss right? Well, it is not that simple. That is a conclusion Aunt Ruchi would make. Think deeper.

Functionally, exercise is very important for us to strengthen our muscles, improve our health, better our endurance and performance at tasks. It is way different if we look at it at a macro level and are typically not just concerned with calories. Infact this is just my level of thinking. Exercise has more than a ton of benefits as you must know. But our concern is to put the spotlight on where it matters most.

If we were just concerned about calories, the whole world would do just 1 form of exercise, the one that burns the most calories, let's say skipping and sprinting (2 of the highest). But that is not the case and that is why when you compare an experienced Yogi vs a Crossfitter or A powerlifter vs a Boxer or a Bodybuilder vs a High-Performance Long Distance Runner. They all look different. Fit, but differently "fit". Nuance helps comprehend this.

What kind of body do you reckon with the most? What do you think would suit you? You be the judge, not anyone, again, not any damn person.

Bodies are a result of the stimulus that they are given. This is the exact reason why they look different. Think broader, question things. Exercise is not just exercise, your body will be the result of the type of exercise you do and do repeatedly.

Now I am not a yoga expert or an expert in any one sort of training method, there are "professionals" for this. But as a generally knowledgeable population, who has time to look at memes, you should know what these forms of training entail when we hear their name. At the very least you must have the cognizance of knowing more or researching when you hear of a new training method or before you let your body undergo that torture. A welcome torture as I'd call it. I would expect you to know that dumbbells and Yoga will not go in the same sentence for example. Or the fact that there are no machines used in Zumba. But fret not, there are thousands of training methods, the only way you know about them is through curiosity. But tracing their origins and underlining some key concepts will take us a long way.

I was blown away when I got to know that I could change the way I look by doing a certain form of exercise rather than what was being taught to newbies at the gym. Post the weight loss, I had lost a lot of muscle and had real big gaps in my body that needed to be filled. I wanted a structured, well built, filled up, hunky body. "Lift heavy weights for lesser reps" somebody at the gym told me. "Do light weights for as many reps as possible" another one told me. "You have to do cardio first, 3 sets of all the machines and then just eat more protein, you will be sorted" another one told. By this time I knew better than to hear them, I nodded along and stuck to doing " my workout plan" I got off of YouTube. Insanely stupid thing to do, but we all make mistakes.

What I was actually training for was to look like a scrawny dude who looks like an amoeba. No shape. So naturally, I dug up google, saw the length and breadth of "exercise science", watched and heard interviews, podcasts and read a ton of articles. I searched up routines of people who I thought I'd want to look like (bad idea I'd never recommend, I stopped this very soon) and I did this for a good time until I could categorise all of exercise known to the 21ˢᵗ century person. Key word, categorize. I think at this point your understanding of these topics clearly decides whether or not you can dig deeper along with me in the further chapters and have a dream body of your own. Read the next few sentences carefully.

I took a 360 degree approach to exhaust all possible exercise or training methods.

To give you some context, some folks would bucket it in these ways:

"Cardiovascular and Muscular"/"Aerobic and Anaerobic"/ "Strength and cardio" and so on. No harm done. All right in their own regard. I went a bit deeper to what I thought was most exhaustive. So exhaustive that I don't leave anything out.

Broadly speaking, I would bucket exercise or activity into these 4. Explained in layman terms

I call it - "The Big 4". This short phrase can help you remember this postulation.

The Big 4:

1. **Aerobic:** Main work here is done by the lungs and heart. Air (oxygen mainly) is a key part of this. Usually done in moderation and for long durations of time. Energy is drawn from oxygen to do this form of exercise.

Function: Get the heart pumping more blood. Pulses racing. Faster breathing.

People call it: Cardio/Cardiovascular training.

Example: Running/Swimming/Walking/Elliptical/Aerobics or cross-trainer type machines found in gyms. Golf, slow walking, not so much. That is normal activity.

2. **Resistance:** Main work done by muscles. Stored glucose - called glycogen present in your body is the energy source for you to be able to do this. The word "Resisit" itself is self-explanatory.

Function: Build endurance, build strength, size (in cases) and power.

People call it: Anaerobic Training/Strength training.

Example: Weightlifting, Powerlifting, Crossfit.

3. **Stability/Balance:** Helps wilfully control and stabilise body position. Helps maintain the centre of gravity. Opens up the body to all sorts of movements. Strengthens the core.

Function: Performance, endurance, athleticism, avoiding injury, recovery from injury.

People call it: No colloquial name.

Example: Pilates, Functional Training, A part of Calisthenics (calisthenics involves mostly bodyweight movements).

4. **Flexibility:** Movement of muscles and tendons. It's self-explanatory here again. It is what the word says.

Function: Avoids fatigue, reduces pain, injury. Increases muscle tolerance. Makes daily activity easier.

People call it: Stretching/Warm up or opening up.

Example: Yoga and its related forms. Hip openers. Stretches of all kinds.

Sure, there are so many forms that prop up nowadays. You name it, they all fall in at least one if not more of these categories. It is not mutually exclusive. But for us. Me and you. Do we need to know more about how an athlete trains? Heck no. Some purists might argue and fight but I am not Michael, to each his own. Some people cannot stand simplicity. This is as easy as I can make it. We will look at the main ones and delineate them in the future chapters to get you to clearly understand what they do your body and how they can be incorporated to achieve your body of choice, but as of now, we can sit back and say pretty confidently, that at a practical level, your thoughts on exercise are not the same anymore. Do yourselves a favour, do not do exercise for exercise's sake. DO NOT EVER COPY/START DOING BLUEPRINTED EXERCISES MADE AND GIVEN OUT OF THIN AIR, without questioning what they are doing to your body. Look for long term sustenance, something that you'd do when you're 60. I suggest everybody look at it that way. We will for sure uncover deeper secrets and micro optimise but mostly, you need to circle back and fixate it. Mostly what mainstream exercise broadly is, has been covered 'The Big 4'. Key word, mainstream.

So, PLEASE UNDERSTAND WHAT HAPPENS WHEN YOU EXERCISE.

EXERCISE: Activity Clock!

Make a note of this on your mobile or on paper!

In a typical day:

> How many hours you sit.

> How many hours you stand/walk doing regular activity.

> How many minutes or hours you spend doing focused exercise/workout.

> How many hours you spend sleeping.

> How many hours do you keep for yourself (self-care, skin care, personal development meditation/therapy and the like)

> How many empty hours do you have (mindless activity/ commute/cooking/errands)

This is what I call your activity clock. Eyeball it, approximate it, but try and guesstimate. The revelations in this are crazy.

Mine for example is - 10:2:1:8:1:2

CHAPTER 5

WEIGHT SCIENCE

Demystifying one of the most googled questions in the world.

**Scene: Me, Michael and the gang were talking about how MMA fighters have to drop kilos of weight to make the weight or qualify for the fight category.**

One person says "They take medicines to pass extra weight through stools"

Other replies "It's damn easy, they are on some water reduction drugs that gets rid of all the water in their body

One more says "It is hard but theoretically simple, they don't eat for 2-3 days and they would drop about 5/6 kilos"

Hot baths, sauna, magic pills. Everything was spoken about that day.

These people speak like they have tried this and is piece of cake. Little do they know" Michael to me.

I think at this point I have to quote one of my favourite sayings.

"As to methods, there may be a million and then some, but principles are few. The man who grasps principles can successfully select his own methods. The man who tries methods, ignoring principles, is sure to have trouble."

— Harrington Emerson

I once heard a renowned "dietician" use these words on a social media post: "Do not look at your food as carbs, fat and protein" (i.e macronutrients), make sure you eat an organic (?), healthy and a balanced meal which is not junk and exercise regularly (whatever that means) and you will lose weight. Better yet, she was fully confident being this generalist. I did not know her intention or thought behind this message but she did ramble on about a tangential topic, like how "eating with bare hands" is more nutritious. I am not going to argue with that. But I have to say that it was one of those rare real life LOL moments for me, where I actually in real life chuckled out loud. I am going to go out on a limb and make a claim that I am not afraid to get backlash on. Most dieticians/nutritionists have surface level knowledge, some bookish and theoretical knowledge about food, which is 100% useful in research and exploratory studies but you see this weight loss/weight gain beast is more psychological, it has to do with human behavioural conditioning and lifestyle changes. Things that are far more complicated than we think it is. Which is why, even after speaking and interacting with me and knowing a thing or two about this topic, it is still not easy for my aunt to lose that weight. Same reason why my dad would not even consider the idea of cutting back on some indulgences.

So, without personal experience, they can only guide you with literature they have learnt but can never empathise, or put themselves in your shoes. To be frank, no one will. Hiring a dietician or a trainer is for outlier situations, the best examples would be for a movie star who needs to change looks and appearance, become like a Greek god on an ad-hoc basis or a president/prime minister who just does not have the time. In those situations, their services would be warranted.

This profession has simply not scaled. I do not mean to generalise. There are millions of very good, knowledgeable people out there who will lay out the very same things laid out in this book and more and there's no harm hiring them if you can afford it, not financially, but afford to stay **dependent**. Which is why I stress on learning and equipping to set yourself up for success. The average Joe finds it really tough to just get his questions answered. My god, the lad wants to shed a few pounds because he went overboard on vacation. Let him do it. You must have experienced this first hand, you ask one (beit common or complex) fitness related question and you will find a slew of conflicting, varying answers. Right?

Let me be honest with you. A "diet" or a "workout plan" will get you nowhere. Absolutely, nowhere.

When the concept of the "diet" in itself is flawed, "dieticians/nutritionists" have no USP in the economy. In the scientific discovery and research world, hell yes, we need more of them, but not in the free market. Diets are short term. You can't live on a diet, lifestyles are long term, in fact, habits and education, they are longer-term. In the last bit, you take control. I can safely say that some "fitness professionals/trainers" again, have no clue about macros or micros. Not all, but more than you'd imagine.

Do fitness pros have a market? 100%, but do all normal people, business owners, corporate bros, white collar workers, blue collar workers, me for example, need them? Absolutely not. Losing weight, gaining weight is dead easy. Gaining muscle is dead easy. Losing fat is dead easy. Dead easy, but on paper. Yes, weight, muscle and fat are different concepts, you can find them being used interchangeably which is blasphemy once you know about the subtleties. (more on this later).

Reverse Conditioning the Brain:

We have been socially conditioned to believe that if we "diet" or eat some specific foods or don't eat a list of foods we will lose weight. We have also been conditioned the same way that if we don't workout every day or do a certain type of exercise repeatedly, only then would you keep fit. (My Dad way of thinking) We live in the world of "I need a diet plan" and "I need a workout plan" to get rid of or put on weight. (Kiara way of thinking) I was on the same boat my entire life and so are many. This is the craziest thing going on. At this point, I feel like it is daylight robbery that most people, apart from the experts, learned or self-educated ones know the science behind weight loss or weight gain, especially when we come to understand that this is elementary stuff.

You must have heard this on the grapevine, "She is married to her diet" or "He is married to the gym". Is that the price we need to pay to get results? One day I kind of circled back, thought to myself, "We are the most intelligent species out there and we practically know the answers to any problem anyone may ever throw at us. We have done years of research in this space and I, a fairly educated person, must be able to break it down". You see break it down I did, pretty successfully but later did I realise that this is a mind game more than a numbers and a science game. But let's look at the numbers and science first, because, remember this - it is very simple and it is an undeniable fact. You cannot disprove it. It is exactly how anybody who ever walked this earth either gains, loses or maintains his or her weight.

For the purposes of lucid understanding of the science of weight loss, we will befriend our old enemy, "the calorie". We will have to do this again and again till he becomes our BFF. He is not that bad actually.

Recalling a formula that you read before;

A - B = ± C, where A is how much you are eating (calories), B is how much you are burning (calories), and C is the value of the difference, which is your current body weight being added or subtracted on a daily basis. It may not be 100% factual, but its a game changer, if you start thinking of your life this way.

A short, 5'4 man may be 110 kilos and fat, a tall, 6'4 man may be a 110 kilos and fit.

Yes, just because one weighs 110 kilos doesn't mean he/she is overweight or fat. Height and muscle mass (more so) are huge factors that determine weight as the bigger person simply has more real estate in the body. This is just one of the million reasons why the weighing scale is not the best determinant of your physical external appearance.

Let's get one thing clear, the quantum of food energy used by an individual (B) changes according to some characteristics such as height, weight, age and our activity habits (mainly). Genetics (rarely). Everybody has a different B value. And obviously, everybody has a different A value (what they ate and in what quantity throughout the day). What your meals were vs what your best friend's meals were today are most likely different. This means C is also different. Again, A- B = ± C

A Thought on Genetics and the Lucky People:

Variable B has one exception however, people with crazy good stars or genetics. Metabolically gifted fellows. Their B is always high. But the catch is, this doesn't last all their life. If they play with biology and defy math, they will end up gaining weight or become "skinny fat". Some people get away with eating anything? Well, no, long term things come to bite them as well. They are doomed. Time is the biggest equaliser.

A classic example here is My Dad, Aunt Ruchi in their 20s-40s, literally ate anything and everything, looked fairly fit. Now, clearly not the case. Matt le Blanc (Joey from FRIENDS) today vs 1999 is another perfect example. Many more examples themselves will present to you when you finish reading the book. These maybe in your public or private life. The math does not differentiate. A - B = ± C

Building towards the weight formula.

BMI:

The BMI or the Body Mass Index is something that haunted me all my life. This is because this godforsaken report always read "obese". Funny times. Why did I get this report? Well, the BMI was and still unfairly is the barometer to determine the "healthy weight of a person". It's everywhere. Many fitness experts rely on it. Strictly do not trust it as it misses out on accounting for many things and differentiating between 2 big things - fat and muscle, which is humongous. I had to mention this as a lot of people, trainers and doctors still, yes in this age, still use this method to opine on your physical state. Even scientists have taken cognizance of this fact and have improved and continue to improve the model.

Hence, the concept of the more colloquial BMI should go out the window. On a BMI scale, you would find the 6'4, 110 kilo man "overweight". You will not believe it but, Phil Heath, Multiple time Mr Olympia winner (World's Most Renowned Bodybuilding Show), probably one of the fittest people on planet earth would be classified as "obese" under BMI. But BMI is used all over. Part of the noise that surrounds the industry. You might have come across this term, almost every gym has a BMI calculating machine. A simple google on the "accuracy of BMI" would really put things in perspective. In simple terms, it is really shady.

The Concept of the BMR:

BMR expands as Basal Metabolic Rate. One will need a certain amount of "energy" or calories or "A" as we learned to just "survive" and lay still or at rest for 24 hours. Let's call it the energy required for your body to just function, internal organs to work and not eat into itself. This is what we call basal metabolic rate (different for each human). In other words this can be represented in calorie values that signify the calories that you need to consume to be able to do biological functions and "just be able to live at rest". You have devices and advanced methods to find this out but we will greatly be benefited with just learning a few methods that eyeball them or closely approximate them and give us a calorie figure, yes calorie figure. (Calories = energy remember?). Some also call this "resting calories"

TDEE – Total Daily Energy Expenditure:

When BMR is the total calories you need to function at rest, TDEE or Total Daily Energy Expenditure is BMR but with activity added in. Or, TDEE is BMR adjusted for activity. Assuming you are a normal human with an eventful life, some duties and hobbies to do, you'd be spending some energy. One of these hobbies may be working out (activity). In short, TDEE gives you the total calories you should be consuming to be able to maintain your weight "given your current lifestyle and existence". This will be called your maintenance calories. Every single human being on this earth has his or her respective "maintenance calories". If you weigh 48 kg and are 5ft 3 and are an athlete, you have a maintenance calorie figure. If you weigh 76 kg and are 5ft 9 and have an office job you have a maintenance calorie figure. A bodybuilder has one, a homeless person has one. But each will be different of course as A, B, C values are different as we garnered. It's important to register this once more, You are not the same as another person, not by a long shot. A, B, C, age, health conditions, this, that and a million things differ from person to person. But, you have a TDEE. That's it, that's the point. Sometimes, this is referred to as maintenance calories.

As a matter of fact, stop what you are doing right now, whoever you are, whether you knew about this or not, it doesn't hurt, go google "Calculate my TDEE" and "Calculate my BMR" and check it right away. This will give you a lot of context with respect to what you are about to read.

The science of weight loss and weight gain is what I have termed as THE WEIGHT FORMULA. Even though it is not just a single formula, the whole concept in itself is pivotal.

The Weight Formula

Maintenance Calories:

Eat at maintenance calorie level and you will maintain your weight. This happens as your energy balance is not being altered. This is your TDEE.

Simple terms: Calories in = Calories out = Maintain weight or Hover around a small range of weight.

Caloric Deficit:

Deficit is creating a small subtraction in energy by reducing calories from the maintenance level. This is either by doing more activity (burning calories), or eating lesser. In essence, altering the body's energy balance. Yes, deficit can be created in 2 ways. Here, your body is receiving less than it burns doing everyday activity. This is the ONLY way to lose body weight. You eat more than you burn, then the body is not losing weight anymore.

Simple terms: Calories in < Calories out = Weight Loss

And if you did not gather,

Caloric Surplus:

Surplus is creating a small addition in energy by increasing calories and altering energy balance. There is only one way to do it and it is to eat more (or inject haha). Here, your body is receiving more than it burns doing everyday activity. This is the only way to gain body weight. You eat more than you burn, then the body gains weight. It's simple addition. Well what kind of weight, important to ask, is something that you will glean very soon.

Simple terms: Calories in > Calories out = Weight gain.

Usual types of weight gain would be;

1) Following a goal-oriented diet and doing rigorous resistance exercise. Calories in > Calories out = Weight Gain (including muscle gain).

2) Over a long duration, eating more than you burn and bam, one day, you see that tire in the mirror or that double chin. (Or that athletic person in high school just lost his high school jawline and abs and now has a beer belly after 7 years of riding on his stars). Everything can be explained.

Now, let's exemplify the equation. (1 kilogram = 2.2lbs = 7,700 calories)

For example, if a man's TDEE shows up to be 2000 calories a day.

1)   GOAL: Weight loss

Maintenance: 2000

Deficit for example (Either by exercise or eating less): 200 (eating 100 calories less and burning 100 calories on the treadmill)

Days to lose a kg: 38.5 (Approx. 1 month and 1 week)

2)   GOAL: Weight Gain

Maintenance: 2000

Surplus for example (Here, eating more only): 400

Days to gain a kg: 19.25 (Approx. 3 weeks or less)

Taking the value of 7,700 Calories = 1 kg. If you look after yourself, create a deficit of 7700 and you would have lost a kg. That is how anybody ever lost a kg. Same way, you slack off or in the odd case you want to gain weight, that's how you do it.

The math is insanely simple, the psychology and practicality of it all is simply not, that is why losing weight is one of the most searched queries on Google.

The understanding of The Weight Formula means, the lucid understanding of the concepts of calorie surplus, calorie deficit and calorie maintenance. It is not rocket science nor is it a new innovation. It is a prerequisite to an effortlessly fit life. Just like how understanding language makes communication easier, understanding the macro math makes physical life and its quality, much easier.

1 + 1 is always 2, it's not debatable. This is called energy balance. This is THE WEIGHT FORMULA. No debates here. This is why it pisses me off, and post today, it should piss you off too when people say "drink green tea to lose weight", "try this juice cleanse and lose weight" it is scientifically not possible. I cannot stress on how many times I have told people this. Aunt Ruchi's Ayurvedic "Kashayam" in the morning filled with honey is a calorie filled carb load no one needs while struggling to lose a couple of kilos. But, according to her, it will help "burn fat from her double chin". Seriously.

"Drink Apple Cider Vinegar, you will lose weight", "Eat lemon zest mixed with cucumber and mint and you'll lose your tummy fat" (No that's not made up, people make up weirder things). I have heard many, I know for sure, you have too. Granted, some of these ingredients may have amazing nutritional and health benefits but NO, they are not black magic. They are food and that is it, for the body, it's just energy. Data. It does not discriminate and pardon those calories. You, as of now, know more than anyone about the concept of what we eat and why exactly we do it.

Let's say your maintenance calories is 2000. If you drink 2100 calories of just "Slim Tea" you will gain weight. Or, you eat 2000 calories of any type of food and 100 calories of "Slim Tea" you will, by all costs, in sometime, gain weight.

Similarly, you can lose weight just by eating cheetos or potato chips in a deficit, burgers and pizza in a deficit and so on. (this is not optimal)

Let's say that your maintenance calories is 1600. If you maintain an average of 1400 by eating just Cheetos, the scale has to go down after a period of time. Or if you are eating 1200 calories of food and 200 calories worth of ice cream every day then at the point where the deficit reaches 7700, a kilo has to drop. There's no arguing this. That is it, task done, mission accomplished right? Just by rereading the book up until here will make you the master of being at your dream weight. You learnt why you eat, you learnt what exactly you eat, you learnt activity and you learnt that activity mixed with the weight loss formula in itself can give you tremendous powers of being able to do anything with your weight.

"Hey, so simple, so I'll just cut my calories by counting what I eat, so I will lose weight, or on the opposite, I'll just increase my calories and I'll gain weight". That would be a daft thing to do. This is a Kiara approach; such a person would be happy to close the book right here and start applying these methods as soon as possible. To them I'd say, hold your horses.

Sure, you will be able to command what weight you would walk around in. But will you master the art of accentuating your look? No. Losing weight is not enough. See, you can be your dream weight and still be unstructured, fat, disproportionate. Let me put it this way, losing or gaining weight will be 80% of your task. Overtime, you will re-read the concepts learnt up until now and master it. Granted. We also agreed that this is highly elementary. Granted again. So, you will be able to do just fine with weight management. You put on a few pounds and you will be able to reduce it. But is that enough? What will give you the edge? How is this different from downloading a fitness app or hiring a fitness coach? The answer is the fact that you will dig deeper and go beyond into the visceral part of the topic.

For starters, learning of the fact that weight is not just weight. Just like we figured out that food was not just food.

EXERCISE: Calorie counting!

> Figure out your TDEE daily/weekly

> Choose an option: maintain/lose/gain

> You are not dieting, just do what you were doing, eat what you were eating.

> Enter everything that you eat into a calorie tracking app, don't worry, over time you will figure out how to use the app better

> Do this for one week, compare the initial data points (TDEE) to the latest ones on the app daily/weekly

CHAPTER 6

"IT'S NOT JUST WEIGHT GODDAMNIT"

Why you didn't gain or lose weight and how this info will drastically change the usage of the word?

Kiara: "You looked way too pale and weak, now you look healthy, your overall size is getting bigger, arms are bigger. Are you gaining weight? You can't tell if someone did not know you" I had actually. But not just weight.

Me: I am bulking. Aiming to get bigger and ill up a bit.

Kiara: What? You want to get fat again? Why would you want to do that? You worked hard Chirag.

Me: "The objective is to optimise for maximum muscle mass and minimum fat percentage taking into account one's short-medium-long term fitness goals and lifestyle"

Kiara: Whatever dude, just don't gain weight again. I can't imagine you being that way.

Me: Don't worry, you will never be witness to it.

Have you ever asked yourself this? In the normal usage of the terms "weight gain" and "weight loss", what weight exactly are we talking about? Where is this magical weight in the body appearing and disappearing from? Have you also observed that weight and fat as terms are used interchangeably?

Here is a way to go about it. You see, weight is not just weight, but it is either water, fat or muscle. Sometimes all 3. Just like food is not just food but it is PCF. Sometimes all 3.

Before you learn anything about physical fitness, you need to question the very basis of appearance. What gives your body its structure? Really, what is it made of? To answer this, I suggest take the peel off approach.

If you peel the human body off layer by layer, just like you would an onion, you will have your answer. This is a schoolboy way of thinking about it. From inside to outside, I have the Skeleton, then the muscles covering it. The skin being the last layer obviously. More study on this and I realised water and fat also constitute the body. The skeleton and skin are not controllable. After you are post pubescent, they stop growing and/or undergoing huge voluntary changes. Muscle, fat and water are however, controllable. **The percentage of muscle-fat-water you have in simple terms is what I call - Body Composition.** You can alter the body composition and yet stay the same weight. That is the power of body composition and that is the weakness of the weighing scale.

So no, your kidneys did not shrink when you lost 5 kilos, and no your liver did not grow in size when you put on 5 kilos either. What was lost or gained was either fat or muscle for the most part. So many people (myself included for the longest time) are just concerned, worried and interested in just the concept of "weight" and nothing else. It is the be all and end all. Let me tell you this, weight and the weighing scale should never be our main concern.

Rewire your brain to ask "What kind of weight am I losing or gaining?" instead of "I just got fat" or "I just need to slim down". Also, please make a habit of regularly checking your weight. Don't wait for someone else or the mirror to let you know your weight. This will lead you to wonderful breakthroughs in your fitness life. I can clearly say that it has changed the way Kiara perceives the term "weight", in whatever context. The answer to that sudden gain will either be fat or muscle. Concerning if it is fat. Good if it is muscle as it is a very tough thing to do. But the sneaky part here is it could sometimes just be water. The most common occurrence of "I gained weight" is fat and water. This is because, over a short duration of slacking off, (considering you are not training with the objective of building muscle and succeeding at it) you simply won't gain muscle so quickly and easily out of thin air. In fact, there is a higher probability that you lost some muscle. Quarantine weight gain? Mini vacation weight? Went bonkers on a holiday weekend? You gained a bit of fat or water weight. Unaccounted weight gained over a long duration will mostly be fat.

Well there you go; weight isn't a concern. You know what is.

Fat and muscle are not new buzzwords that I have presented. It is an extension to what you have already read. They are closely, very closely related to **PCF** and the **The Big 4**. Something that you are well equipped to understand at this point. Ergo, I say that our objective is to keep that muscle level high or in the worst case not lose it, and keep the fat level or percentage of the body that is fat, low. The lesser the fat content in your body the better it is.

The Usual Calorie Surplus Scenarios:

1) Take this, if you have mini spurts of surplus calories, (duration of hours or very few days), then most of this extra "weight" is stored in your liver and muscles as glycogen (stored glucose). That's it. Can't grasp it? Screw it, I just brought that up to make a point in context. This glycogen is not all that bad. This is what happens after you went overboard with that dinner buffet. This is good energy that can be used for doing strenuous work in the near future.

2) But, an elongated surplus (what happened to my dad or aunt ruchi over the years) results in fat stored in adipose tissue all around your body.

3) An even longer but bigger surplus means worse things to the body, huge amounts of weight gained and sometimes leading to a medical condition in obesity. So now you know biologically, how the fattest person you know got fat. That is all the science you need to know. Basically, fat spreads all around the body and has a tendency to settle right below our skin, that is where the adipose tissue is located

(4th grade bell rings again), that is why you get flabby, your waist size increases, so on and so forth.

You cannot dictate where and how you store this "extra meat". Likewise you simply cannot select spots to reduce them from. Hankerings like "I want to reduce face fat", "I want to reduce abdomen fat" or "I want to reduce buttock fat'' are not a possibility. I suggest you go to whatever lengths to etch the last sentence in your brain. This is called "spot reduction". And spot reduction is simply not possible. There are workarounds to make body parts look better but I repeat, spot reduction of fat is not possible. Everybody has that "one place" where they accumulate a lot of fat. That one place that is the first victim. For most it is the abdominal area, although I have seen people complain about the same with their chest, lower back and surprisingly face. Nobody likes a double chin or a ballooned up face, I guess. But I am sorry, the obstacle of spot reduction has simply not been broken down yet. Even after years of iterations by so many experts in the field.

Notice one thing here. It is not fat, **the macronutrient** that makes us fat but **food in surplus** that makes us fat. Read the last sentence at least 5 times. I tell you this because we as a society are marketed that fat the macronutrient is bad. Sure, it has 9 calories, but no, not 1 single macro ever made anybody fat. It's the surplus. Even if you knew about it. It is always nice to ping our brain about that again. The macronutrient fat and the fat that you are gaining are two different things. And that is why weight and fat are not the same. That is aunt Ruchi level thinking. We established that eating broccoli in a surplus will also make you "fat". It is just difficult and far fetched but that is still possible. This clearly solves one of the world's most misunderstood things - "eating high-fat (the macronutrient) food makes you fat". People for years have steered away from cheese, butter, nuts, healthy oils and other fat rich food. The free market i.e. the thriving food companies, pseudo experts, your own brain will tell you to stay away from fat. Fat is not the problem. Fat doesn't make you fat. Excess calories does. Not a single fat free product does anything special. Not a thing, zilch. I repeat, do not abstain from high fat foods because they are bad. This is just one of the re-wirings you need to do to your system before claiming your nutritional freedom. Clearly, this is not the case and you will yourself learn that fat the macronutrient is not our enemy at all. It can be, under circumstances, your very best friend to reduce the amount of fat percentage in your body. This is called ketosis (something you might have heard about already) which we will soon learn and evaluate at depth.

"Weight is not the matter but fat and muscle are. Makes sense, but how do I control fat% and muscle mass in the body?"

The answer to that is nothing new to you, it comes down to what I call stimulus. It comes down to: I'd explain it this way to my dad;

1. Playing around with how you work out or do activity

2. Playing around with how you eat

Okay, we cannot afford to stay ambiguous anymore. It's time we get to the meat. I'd say this to Michael;

1. Optimising your exercise/The Big 4

2. And optimising your macros/PCF

Your physical self is the result of how good these 2 points are handled in the long run. For now, some of you might be milking your genetic stars, or some of you might be wondering where things went wrong, but in the long run, have some sort of control over these 2 things and you are 100% on the way to nutritional and fitness freedom. For those of you who are "thin" and young, remember, we don't want you being Aunt Ruchis and Matt Le

Blancs of the world. For those of you who are overweight, fat or looking to get catapulted, these 2 i.e., getting the right training in, getting in the right food in the right macronutrient proportions or macro splits known colloquially will be of paramount importance. Food remains food, how much of what you eat changes. Same goes for training, workouts remain workouts, how much of what type of exercise (remember the buckets) you do becomes important. Even if you do not want to become a hulk or go crazy with big shoulders, having a higher concentration of muscle will help in looks, metabolism, strength and longevity.

You cannot gain weight and lose weight out of thin air. If anybody ever lost or gained weight, there was an addition; i.e., Muscle/Fat/Water. Or there was a subtraction, i.e., Muscle/Fat/Water.

You should worry about muscle as that is what gives your body shape and you should worry about fat as that is what takes it out of shape.

Connection with Metabolism:

If you can recall, I had renamed metabolism as absorption when I first learnt it. Absorption can be called using up of calories. Aerobic exercise burns more calories in the short run - cardio. This is an undeniable fact. Doing more cardio, doing more aerobic exercise, pushing your guts out doing this will lead to more calorie burn. Importance here is on quantity.

Muscle however burns more calories at rest. Yes, you heard that right. Muscle burns calories at rest. When you are not doing anything, because you have more muscle mass, your BMR, TDEE increases. It is simple to understand really. Lions eat more than cats. Let's say Hulk and Hawkeye eat 2400 calories for the day. Hulk is eating in a deficit while Hawk Eye may be eating at maintenance or even surplus. Because of so much real estate in the body, Hulk also guzzles up calories quickly, making his metabolism super fast. This is why you see big dudes eat in volumes. All this is great but building muscle is a long process.

This is your only answer to the question of should I do more cardio or lift more weights. Over the long run, my suggestion is that you concentrate on resistance and muscles. I mean who does not want to sit back and let the body do all the work.

The more muscle you have in your body the more your body requires energy. Register this.

I reiterate - absorption is metabolism. Metabolism is a chemical process that requires energy. Well, there you go, more muscle mass means more metabolic, at least comparatively. Your body simply absorbs more because it needs more. This seriously puts you in a position to get away with a lot of things. A lot. This is not my opinion in any way. This is reality.

Managing Muscle:

"Muscle is built when muscle protein synthesis is greater than the rate of muscle protein breakdown" What again? Did that make sense? Not for me too the first time I read it and multiple folks have turned their back when I say this to them.

So, it makes sense we take a different and easier approach first.

One out of 2 main parts of building and maintaining muscle is exercise, especially resistance training. So, you could be doing yoga or walking for the most time as "your workout" but there, you would just mostly be doing calorie burning. Until your body is faced with resistance and your muscles are not overworked or under some tension, you will not be in a position to activate it let alone to maintain or build it. From an exercise point of view, muscle is built (hypertrophy or anabolic state as Michael would call it) when it is overloaded progressively with resistance, fed with the right protein and given enough rest. The best way to do it - lifting and putting down weights. If not that, adding some or the other form of resistance. Do not get bogged down, you do not have to move a crazy ton of weights if you don't want to. We will not delve into bodybuilding and nerd concepts just yet but just knowing the fact that one should get their body used to resistance with exercise, be it by extra volume (quantum of exercise done), repetitions, actual weight or even intensity is more than enough. That resistance you provide is the sole difference between the muscle mass present in a zumba instructor vs the muscle mass in a person that does "push ups" at home as his daily exercise and that muscle mass of a bodybuilder. This is not to say that non resistance exercises are not good. As The Big 4 suggests, each type of exercise or training has its own benefits. Aerobic exercise helps you burn more calories easily with lesser effort like running. Flexibility and Balance exercises avoid injuries among other things. Strength or resistance exercise takes care of your muscle mass. Which is important and you know why.

The second variable you need to worry about when it comes to muscle is protein. It is protein's chemical and biological effects that speak to the muscles in the body. They are called the building blocks of muscle. This primary school explanation goes a long way for people. While you do resistance training, let's take an example of lifting dumbbells and doing bicep curls, your body undergoes a lot of damage, endures pain. It is protein that makes up for the damage, rebuilds it, time and again. This constant back and forth is what helps muscles grow and it's simply not possible without protein. This happens with all resistance activities, even picking up a heavy grocery bag.

Enough of the mumbo-jumbo, the point is, protein speaks easily with the muscles and vice versa. Look at it this way, for all practical purposes, from a fitness point of view, **muscle only sees protein and strength training, it is blind to everything else**. That is your answer to how any muscular guy you know got that way - he ate more protein and did some resistance type training. You can also make this out in girls. Girls who have more muscle are what you call "toned".

Get this, if you have ever gained weight, it is mostly because of a carbohydrate and fat surplus and definitely, definitely not the cause of the protein surplus. First of all, a protein centric surplus will not make you look fat, it will make you look fuller, muscular obviously and strong and second of all it is ridiculously tough to eat a lot of protein. It's highly satiating.

A thought on satiation and how can you play around with it?

Satiety is the right opposite of hunger. It is the state of being full. It is tough to fill yourself up with carbohydrates, it is easily digestible and the body will keep asking more of it. Protein and fiber (the indigestible carb) however are more satiating, it fills you up to the point of disgust. Compare eating 4 donuts to 4 pieces of chicken breast. Yes, now you know what I'm talking about. The doughnuts just dive right in.

Foods that are lower in weight but high in calories are called calorically dense foods, dense foods more often than not contain fat mixed with carbs, let's not forget one gram of fat is 9 calories. Too much cost for too little reward. **Eg:** 50 grams of highly processed, refined sugar syrup. About 300 calories. Mostly carbs and fat.

Foods low in calorie and high in quantity/weight are called high volume foods. **Eg:** 6 egg whites scrambled. About 100 calories. More than 50g in weight. Mostly protein.

Protein and fiber (remember chapter 2) are known to be satiating. Filling. Hunger killing. 4 plates of chicken salad will actually kill hunger for you more than 2 chicken burgers from McDonald's. Keyword is hunger killing and not satisfying. People chase the latter. Latter being taste. Again this comes back to what your reason for eating food is. And no, I am not suggesting that you never have McDonald's either. Life can be lived. With the McDonald's meal, sure it was tasty but who ever filled their stomach with just two burgers? I want fries and nuggets and everything else on the menu.

In essence you can really eat more (in quantity) to lose weight. Funny how that works out.

Fats are not the enemy, nor are carbs. But excess carbs surely, surely are! I will tell you what is doomsday - excess carbs + fat in a surplus. The density and non satiety in the combo is just a horrible combination.

PROTEIN = SATIETY = NO DEBATE!

Managing Fat:

Unlike muscle management, which had 2 levers, fat can be controlled with only 1 lever. Calorie deficit. Thankfully this can be done in 2 ways which makes it flexible for us. This is the only way to make your body tap into the "fat reserves". There has to be an energy deficit, an imbalance which will force the body to scavenge all places and end up using its own stored fat for energy. This is what people mean by "burning fat".

Approach 1A - (Eat less intelligently): This is to just maintain a calorie deficit. Better if it is a deficit with a higher protein consumption than normal. Cause you know, just eating less will make you look scrawny. Protein digestion in itself is tough which means the body is burning calories due to the load by default. And also, it helps regulates muscle mass which is overall a half decent thing at he very least. When it comes to losing fat or tapping into the fat in the body for energy as I'd like to call it, the energy balance needs to be altered. And that is why the deficit is a MUST.

Approach 1B (Eat less differently): In school and in the earlier parts of the book, we learnt that, after consuming a meal, because of metabolism/absorption (remember chapter 2), the body converts the carbohydrates from your food into energy (glucose) and all excess carbohydrates will be stored as glycogen and then, if left idle, fat (too much of a surplus). What if instead of carbohydrates or protein, fat is the main source of energy for the body, we survive on a fat centric diet, eating foods with a higher percentage of the macronutrient fat in it. Over a long duration, the body starts using fat as fuel (it can be conditioned to do so) and becomes a live fat burning machine. I am again alluding to ketosis, we will learn more about this "not so sustainable" form of diet pretty soon. I do not suggest method 1B for anyone over the long term.

Approach 2 (Controlling Exercise/Training):

Remember, aerobic exercise "burns" more calories than any other alternative. Maintain or increase deficit by burning more calories so that the gap energy that the body is tapping into will be from stored body fat. Some exercises burn more than others. But for now, we know that fat can be managed through approach 1A, approach 1B or Approach 2. Plain and simple.

That is fat and muscle taken care of!

Managing Water

Well just like how 2/3 of the Earth is covered in water, approximately to 2/3 of the human body is also filled with water. Well, that does hold a lot of weight doesn't it. This is often forgotten by the general population.

Water again should be optimal, something I realised was too little water and too much water both are not good. If you have too much water, you will look bloated. If you deplete all the water in the body, you will look amazing. Yes, you read that right. Your body will show it's true, aesthetic, muscular self. Again, nobody other than a bodybuilder wants to see that you may think. But wrong, sometimes, it may help you. I sure have seen some models cut down on the water content in the body before their "photo shoot". Yes, the world is crazy (or not).

We are often guilty of having too much water in the body rather than too little. Sometimes forcing it to do so. Well, other than water being used for the bodily functions, it constantly keeps adjusting itself for the circus that we do thanks to our eating habits. Along with controlling water intake, people also control food to alter the water present in the body.

The next two points will be very, very important for you.

- Per gram of carbohydrate consumed, the body holds about 2 to 3 g of water.

- A slightly divergent but very important point in the context of dieting here - Sodium. Sodium is the mineral that is responsible for regulating water content in the body. sodium is highly present in processed food and salt among other things.

The more spicy, processed, salty food you eat, especially if it is mixed with carbs, you feel bloated this is because of the sudden retention of water that your body is getting used to.

Reducing these 2 factors can also get rid of some, I stress on some, water in the body. This is why people in bodybuilding shows, models prior to shoots or events, deplete almost all the water in the body by reducing water itself, carbohydrates and salt. They stick to sipping water by counting it in drops. Maniacal, yes. But I am nobody to judge. This is called being show ready. Do not attempt this without expert guidance. Infact, do not play with reducing or increasing water and going overboard.

The above paragraphs were written to prove a point, that is that weight is not just weight. It's _______,_______,________. Fill up the blanks yourself.

So yes, if you want a quick trip to town weightloss or rather water loss, reduce carbs and sodium. You would be bloat free. I am kidding, don't ever take short cuts. Try it, see it, but don't swear by it. The objective of this topic is to just be aware that water is a part of your body and that holds weight and it is still controllable through food.

So, just like weight is not weight, but fat, muscle and water, calories are not just calories, a diligent person would also learn more about managing macros as we just figured out there's so much strength the trio of PCF has. For long term freedom in fitness, be it in the form of losing, gaining or maintaining your weight or fitness levels, calorie counting is simply not enough. It is macro counting that will definitely help you get around the rough edges.

EXERCISE: Affirmations to the Rescue!

This is exercise is more a job of the mind. I want you to go to the mirror and tell these 10 affirmations by looking at yourself in the eye and everything as if you mean it.

"Weight does not matter as much as how I look in the mirror"

"Body composition is a better indicator of how you look than weight"

"I want to look good naked"

"Supplements are NOT a must if I have to see substantial results"

"I will not compare my body and looks to anybody else's, I will strive to make this body of mine better than it was yesterday"

"One cannot target where I can lose or gain weight"

"I will make sure I sacrifice 1-2 ours for self and body care"

"I will always cross verify fitness advice I come across anywhere"

"Carbs or any single macronutrient is not the enemy or a friend"

"Weight training does not make you bulky"

"You don't require a written diet or workout plan to lose weight or gain weight"

MORE ON MACROS

Making them your "hedge" against an unfit life.

If you are under the impression that theory is the be all and end all, you are mistaken. As much as this book can help you ease the learning process, practical application in real life is a must to see any result. If I haven't guided you towards practical discovery, then I would have failed. One just cannot understand the complexities of balancing and modifying anything without first hand experience. Same goes for calories, same goes for PCF. One cannot just master the macronutrient intake until you count them, calculate them and manage them. In real life. It might sound geekish, eccentric or even crazy but, the concept of calculating, or being aware, consciously, what goes in your mouth would be the single biggest favour you would have done for yourself. Believe me, a lot of food enters the mouth, dozens of thousands of times in a year. You do not need to do this bizarre thing of counting what you eat life long, that's far from the truth, but, you have to do it, someday. And this someday or days, will not last long. Nobody can stand scrupulously weighing, counting, calculating and messing up their sanity and thereby their entire life. But doing it when matters pays you off.

Concept of Macro Splits:

Fit people eat in macro splits. Knowingly or unknowingly. Macro splits are quite literally the division of macronutrients (in percentage % terms) that one should be eating at every day.

They are expressed usually in the order of PCF. Your total daily calories come from the following macronutrients in that proportion. It could be (P-C-F) 40-40-20 or 50-30-20 or even 25-10-65 or any combination under the sun. But these 3 are popular.

Again, they go in the order of PCF or Protein, Carbohydrates and Fats and their respective percentages.

Here is Michael's: 50-30-20 (high protein diet)

Here is Kiara's: 30-40-20 (balanced but comparatively higher protein diet)

Here is my dad's: 10-70-20 (carb heavy diet - vegetarian)

Here is Aunt Ruchi's: 20-60-20 (non-vegetarian but carb heavy still)

Carbs Are a Majority in Most People's Macro Split:

Fact of the matter is that we all seem to have a predominantly carbohydrate heavy diet. There is no denying it. They are accessible, cheap and tasty. But they are what I call, "just a bit too sketchy". The process of carbohydrate metabolism, something like carbs digest into glucose that is stored as glycogen, blah blah blah, all takes place in the presence of Insulin. Simply put, carbs can be converted into energy only and only under the presence of insulin which is a human produced hormone, something every normal human has. The next part gets interesting.

This overeating of carbs, thereby leading to more active glucose in the body is the definition of diabetes. Because you have glucose, your body needs insulin and starts producing more of it, this gets more and more and boom one day, you are not only in bad shape but you have diabetes, most obese people are diabetic. This is why diabetics take insulin shots. Their body simply needs that much insulin. Much beyond what a normal body can produce. The body's ability to regulate insulin goes for a toss.

This is type 2 diabetes - found in people due to obesity and food abuse. Type 1 diabetes is a medical condition that is unavoidable for some. Higher glucose is the enemy in either case.

Available in abundance, addictive, silent killer type characteristics. Smoking? No, carbs. This is why carbs are hated by the fitness community and the food industry each and every day has a higher demand for carbs. We are producing, processing and eating more carbs than ever. This generation will go down in history as a generation with great tolerance towards carbs. Our ancestors did not simply eat so much of carbs as they; 1. Had better things to do than process food, 2. Ate meat by hunting and killing. But the thing is, you can change your body to get "less used" to carbs. The trick is being malleable enough to unlearn.

The Macro SPLIT in Reality:

Let us exemplify the macro split. If hypothetically Michael's maintenance calories is 2,400 and his macro split is 50-30-20. Remember, this maintains his weight. Then;

50% of his calories come from Protein = 1200 calories (50% of 2400)

– therefore, he eats 300 grams of Protein (1 gram of protein = 4 calories, 300 x 4 = 1200),

30% of his calories come from carbs = 720 calories (30% of 2400)

– therefore, he eats 180 grams of carbohydrates (1 gram of carbohydrate = 4 calories, 180 x 4 = 720)

20% of his calories come from fat = 480 calories (20% of 2400)

– therefore, he eats approx 50 grams of fat (1 gram of fat = 9 calories, 50 x 9 = 450 rounded off).

(And he is a vegan, wow)

He now has to just pick and eat foods that get him as close to the 300 gram protein mark (that is way too much and not easy, take it for what it is = an example), 180 gram carbohydrate mark and 50 grams fat mark. Stress on as close to. I know this is overwhelming. I don't want anybody to go as deep unless they are looking for some laser sharp results. Even having cognizance of these facts, getting as close as possible is way more than enough. This knowledge will only help you during tougher times.

Do the same exercise of counting macros, creating splits and finding out quantity in grams for all the others and go one step ahead, take your maintenance calories and pick a macro split and try for yourself. Do it once, and don't ever do it again, most people don't have to. But doing once goes a stupendously long way.

Macro splits are mainly important for goals. Just knowing your calorie stuff and increasing or decreasing may help you in understanding weight loss/weight gain science but it is the macros that matter for the fat and muscle as we figured out. Macro splits help you adhere to rules and get the body reacting to how you want it to react. Following a 40-40-20 split during your weightloss might just help you hold on to some muscle mass rather than just picking a deficit and going for it blindly. There is an ocean of a difference between a person who just knows the concept of weight science or The Weight Formula (deficit and surplus) vs a person who knows macros (atleast in theory). All diets should be made on the basis of macro splits and macro counting.

We will dig deep into playing with macros soon and knowing this will be of the greatest of help to you. When I told you that the concept of macros is the most important in the book I wasn't kidding. The past few paragraphs are an exercise of a lifetime. This is the base to what I call my version of "Flexible Dieting Lifestyle". FDL or flexible dieting lifestyle is a hidden gem that helps people be nutritionally free. But over the years I have mastered it and put my own twist to it instead of renaming it, I want all of you to stick to the term "Flexible Dieting Lifestyle" or FDL in short.

When speaking to people like Michael, "macros" has a very advanced meaning. Commonly, this is how it goes down.

Q - "Hey man, what are your macros right now?"

A - " I'm looking at 150P 280C 60F for now" – Micheal

– Macros are PCF, up until chapter 5 you (well most of you)

"How do you count and track calories/macros? This seems to be a nightmare."

Other than the fact that you know the macro food chart and the calories each macro has (449), you need nothing else. But really, a food measuring scale and an app goes a long way unless you can eyeball and are good with weight measurement by the hand (I am kidding of course). The food measuring/weighing scale to weigh the food, and an app to double track and stay accountable. Tons of such apps exist with millions of food data that tells you the PCF value for anything. It is the most efficient way. The apps in the market have tons of features too. Just log or enter what you ate, the app shows you total calories, macros, daily macro splits, weekly, monthly data for the same. You can also set a deficit or surplus calories as these apps also calculate your TDEE. It's really all in one.

All you need to be careful of is entering the right dish (or the closest dish that you can find that's similar) and be aware of the quantity. There are bar codes for packaged foods as well. Software and tech I believe, has really helped this industry. For a restaurant example, if you are having a pepperoni pizza, type a 11 inch pepperoni pizza with and it's highly likely you'd find the item in the app. If not, just enter a margarita pizza and add pepperoni or any other topping you had. Both get the job done. This is the pizza example, do the same for other dishes. Either log in as it is, or break them down and enter the constituent parts in its approximate quantities. After a dedicating period of time doing this, there is no one catching you. Pretty soon, you can ballpark the calories and macros of any dish in any restaurant.

Great, you mean to say that I need to carry a food measuring scale and make some precious space in my phone for a macro calculating app that I have to use after every meal?

Yes and No. Do not worry, as a normal person, who has tons of better things to do than to sit and count calories first of all, forget macros. Believe me, I was there too and at this point I do not count all macros. Nor do many advanced fitness experts. This is because not only can I do it mentally, but in the long run, protein and total calories is all that matters for people even in the intermediate stage (been a really fit person for >3 years consistently). I still do get fidgety and ultra track food when I slack off, key is, when I slack off. You will not believe how much we sneak into our pie holes. Tracking works brilliantly if you are looking for serious results.

Eventually, no one will ever track forever. Simply LONG TERM UNSUSTAINABLE. But to get to a level of comfort, a short sample of time has to be dedicated towards counting calories and all macros. You can pick your time and align it however. Maybe you have a wedding coming up, maybe you always wanted to lose that tyre on your stomach or maybe you do not have any motivation at all. Just do it. Kiara did it to get ready for her graduation. Irrespective of the reason, those 60 days were life changing for her. Consider 1-2 months of calorie and macro counting as summer camp and do it. This habit compounds very well. Do it diligently and your thinking about food will change forever. Once this is done, if it is working out for you, continue it, if not you would have learnt so much. My belief is not everyone can or has to do it long term. Not even insane food geeks cannot afford to do it every day. They just do it during times of need. I do as well during times of need. 80% of the year I do not even look at calories. I just eat intuitively. Most fit people do this. But the hard work put in that short period of time makes all the difference. It is that effortless if you put yourself to it and ride the wave of the class that is "macro counting". It is almost like cheating. Fit people have cravings too, fit people eat junk too. They don't just burn it off but they are better off because they know how macros work (they counted) and how they can adjust their days around those cheat meals. Trust me when I say this. It surely pays off, but it is also a pain in the ass. You picked this book up to really get to the bottom of the subtitle, you will by all means get there but macros are a huge stop in this train journey. JUST DO IT!

I repeat, after you have done it (gone through the process of macro counting, playing with splits for a fair amount of time) and it is second nature to you, all you need to worry is about the fundamentals. Protein, training and overall calories are what you should be concerned with, in the LONG RUN. Post some really good (and bad) experiences going to gurus, turning to "influencers", reading a ton on these topics, I learnt this and I will keep repeating this to myself.

"Other than bones and organs, my body is either water, muscle or fat." That is it and the best part is all these 3 are tractable. Tractable through macros, tractable through training"

There is no stopping anybody who has deeply ingrained this concept. He/She can be fit or fat. At will. It becomes a literal game. We went from "What to do now, I need to become fit or lose weight" on page 1 to exactly knowing "What weight you gained in the first place, is it something that you should be worried about in the short term (could be water), in the long term (elongated surplus that added up all these years) and in either case, what exactly you should do to reverse the situation and get to achieving what you want!"

EXERCISE: Macro Counting!

This is just like how you counted calories the last time around. This time you are counting macros.

> Pick up a macro split 40:40:20/50:30:20/33:33:34 whatever.

> And then macros (something on the lines of 150P:100C:50F)

> Decide your foods, enter everything in the app and try and get as close as possible to hitting your macros

> Do this for 5 days-one week, if you have done this already before, 2x your time

Take a look at all the food you eat and compare this to the original diet that you made **on chapter 1**

CHAPTER 7

THE DIETING ZOO!

How to do away with the concept of "diet"!

My dad: "Chirag, I know you follow this western way of eating. It's not good for you"

Me: What?

My dad: You keep telling things about keto and you don't eat in the morning and added to that I see you experiment with your body too much"

Me: No dad it is not like that.

Him: Just eat a normal vegetarian diet like us and you'll be healthy. I heard my colleague try this nut based diet and he fell sick for a week.

Me: Sure dad!

This is a psychological game, something deep rooted in your system. Altering things like habits, body composition, cravings, taste, innate wants and needs it's not a short term thing. Chase lifestyles and not short-term cash courses.

If I can mark the trajectory of the best and the most fittest people I know, professionals or otherwise, people who stay fit year round, there is one glaring pattern. They first build up the requisite subject matter knowledge, then, they do away with trainers and dieticians, then, give up following a rigid workout plan/routine or a diet plan. Sure, they do plan for some specific short term goals but it will be 100% self made with the help of research, how it helps them with their goals and applying sound logic. An example of a goal here is maybe building up some muscle mass for a feeble looking guy. For which you know what steps they'd take; up protein intake, include big time resistance training and be in a calorie surplus. It is important to mention another type of goal for contrast. Let's assume the goal is to just be 3 kgs less for your wedding day so you'd fit in that suit. Then they'd straight up go on the necessary calorie deficit and focus on cardio/aerobic exercise as this helps burn more calories. Maybe they'd reduce carb intake and sodium intake to drop some water weight if they're clever. These people just manage to fit things into their normal life.

This is your nutritional and fitness freedom. This I believe is a true superpower. Getting to this level takes years of experience and trials and errors. Every chapter that you have read up until now, was months, if not years of learning for these folks.

You may ask, "How do I make my own diet then?", "How do I make my own workout plan?"

We will examine the former in this chapter to get you to GOD level. To answer that question you will need to know how any diet ever came into reality.

Hundreds of millions of people every single day go on a diet. I believe at least 50% of the population of any given point is thinking of going on a diet short or maybe long term. And to help that lunacy, we live in a world of 101 diets. I'm kidding obviously, there are more than that I'm sure. My cynical tone is thanks to months of trying these variations and wasting precious time and mental energy.

Up until now, you have built a deep foundation with respect to food and macros but not dieting. I would not be lying if we all agreed on one fact, at this point you know more theory than tips for actionable use in the kitchen or at the restaurant. That is exactly how one should approach these things. Just practically experimenting every new fad will lead you to a dead end. Each and every time. This is because tips and tactics are like the cherries on top. Fundamental concepts and systems will take you a long way and enable you to employ these tips, tactics and even tricks.

For example: You wouldn't know the implications of carbohydrates holding water in your body (water weight gain), if you didn't know your food contains carbohydrates in the first place (My dad category of thinking). Hence, we go step by step.

We learnt the theory of food, great. But now it's time to take the practical class if you will. In the real world this is called "dieting". This thing has a very negative connotation. I'd like to change it to "eating habits" or "eating patterns". I forced myself to rename the term and you wouldn't believe the sort of changes that I started to see. I stuck to eating patterns/habits whenever I wanted to reference the term "diet". Just giving it a positive spin helps you. Think about it. Now you don't ever need to say to your friend at a party you are "On a diet". How about you say, "I don't have a habit of eating this or that". How about you say "I am trying to eat differently". Half the game is won here.

As suggested, to know how to make your own diets, we will skim through and trace how dieting came to this world in the first place.

The word "Diet" really does not have a solid definition which the majority agrees to. For some, it may mean "something that you do to lose weight" (Aunt Ruchi)

For some it may mean "something that the nutritionist gives you" (my dad)

For some "The thing that keeps you healthy" (a Kiara when she started off)

For bodybuilders like Michael it is a term that they use when they are cutting body fat or getting ready for a vacation. A period of "Rigorous and scrupulous caloric and macro counting"

My definition is that a diet is your individual eating habit or pattern which is subject to change at any given time. Patterns or habits can have one-time deviations, sure, but largely they represent a long term "you". Dieting, on the other hand, is highly "short term". People know this, they have not internalised this yet. That is why you hear "Diet starts from Monday", or "Diet starts after Diwali" etc.

Diets/dieting is a gargantuan thing in the world, it's an industry, a multi-billion dollar one at that. Let's take a scan of the market that gets hideous as we go:

The Zoo and Its Animals.

Paleo

High in protein. No dairy, gluten, grains, soy, or corn.

Carb-Conscious

40-50g net carbs or fewer, with plenty of protein.

Gluten-Free

Wheat alternatives. Not suitable for those with severe gluten allergies.

Lean & Clean

Whole foods with less than 600 calories/serving.

Ketogenic

Less than 30g net carbs, high in fat.

Vegetarian

No meat or seafood.

Pescatarian

No meat or poultry. Vegetarian meals + seafood.

Mediterranean

Whole grains, good fats, seafood and responsibly sourced meats.

Carnivore

No plants, just meat.

Vegan

No meat or dairy, mostly plant based.

Intermittent Fasting:

Not a diet

Given that some here are diets, some are even medical condition based eating, some socio economic movements, some named after regions and whatnot, it is comedic. The clutter that this is, is one of the main reasons most diets don't stick.

These are the prevalent ones. I picked these ones because they propagate themselves or are marketed in a way that proclaims good health, effectiveness in terms of weight loss/fat loss and general well-being. Which is what people allude to when they hear the term.

Eating lesser carbs is a good habit, fasting it's a very good habit, showing less cruelty towards animals it's also a very good cause. But, making it your eating reality until and unless it's not authentic to you, will not fetch you long-term results. It will not be "you". Remember this, you fall into any one of these diet traps and you will never be independent again and forget about your nutritional freedom.

Scanning the market: A slightly deeper look into some of these well known diets. I want to say this, these diets have their own reasons for complexities. They are a branch of study if you will. This is not an encyclopaedia but more so a reference guide.

The Ketogenic Diet:

The science behind the keto diet is fool proof. Remember when I told you food is the only energy known to man. Well in the 21ˢᵗ century body, this energy is mainly from carbohydrates (and a little from protein) which metabolises as glucose > Glycogen > Fat. In the simplest way put, on the keto diet, you devoid your body of glucose or carbohydrates as main source of energy, allowing it to adapt itself into using fat, the macronutrient and its metabolism as fuel and thereby it becomes a virtual fat burning machine. During this "adapting itself" the body turns to the only other fuel it can use - Ketones. Ketones are produced only in the absence of glycogen. It is produced by the liver when there is an absence of insulin is sensed. (Remember: Insulin is a hormone used to convert glucose to energy)

The macro split is something like this:

25%-30% of calories come from Protein

10% or less calories come from Carbohydrates.

65%-70% of calories come from Fat

A 2000 calorie diet would have 150 P 145 F 25 C

(If you're confused, re-read the last chapter)

Easy to read on paper, literal mammoth to do in real life.

The keto diet has rightly gained fame. Incredibly effective in the short run. It is almost like weight loss magic. It starts working from within days and you will drop weight like an MMA fighter two days prior to his fight. Remember, you still have to be in a calorie deficit. Apart from this, the diet has immense biological and medical benefits that go just beyond weight loss. I would recommend anybody to enquire into that at their free time while we stick to the physical effects of the ketogenic diet.

Is this the most effective over the short run? Yes

Is this the most efficient way to lose weight? 100% not.

Would I advise anybody to pick this up other than outlier conditions? Hell no.

If you have picked up this book and have had some sort of experience dieting or experimenting with the diets. You must've come across this infamous, scary astonishingly efficacious Keto diet. A majority of people I know who have followed it including me do not do it for more than 90 days at MAX. I would consider this to be a get rich quick scheme. Can work, but can you do it lifelong? Keto is something that is completely worth it in the short run. Enormous sacrifices, sourcing materials, cooking them, counting each and every macro, judiciously counting carbohydrates, or spending money on somebody for you to do it. This diet screams unsustainability.

Also, we have, in the 21st century, a huge inclination to carbohydrates and carb rich food. And carbs are amazing. I don't want to miss out on my favourite burger and waffles with ice cream on top for a keto diet. I'd do something cleverer.

Well at this point even for the most tried and tested, this remains a FAD. Unless you have been on the keto diet and consuming food in that macro split since birth, it is very tough to get hooked onto. But some folks actually catch on to it and do keto lifelong. Props to them.

Low Carb:

This sort of a diet is very close to keto but not necessarily keto. People over time realised the effects of too much supply of carbohydrates to the body. A low carb diet is a low carb but higher protein diet. It is not a high fat diet like the keto diet.

Macro splits here could be:

50%-60% of calories come from Protein

25%-30% of calories come from Carbohydrates

10%- 15% of calories come from Fat

More sustainable than most diets. You will have to really eat a lot of protein in this which means you will be less hungry always. Sustainable, doable, overall optimal.

Paleo:

The paleo diet is a diet that is the poster child for the word FAD. Here, your foods solely consist of foods available during the palaeolithic era. When was this era specifically? It doesn't matter, they told you it works, remember, so, blinkers on, and follow. Somehow this diet has no information or rules with macros. So, forget trying to achieve anything substantial through this diet. You will plateau really quick (reach a few quick milestones if any and the effectiveness stops).

Truly amazing how we marketed a whole bunch of fanatics about something that existed 2-3 million years ago. To give you a brief, the palaeolithic era did not know anything about processing and modern technology. This means no food that goes into the factory can be consumed, along with many other such palaeolithic concepts. Your typical foods are:

Fruits, Vegetables, Nuts and Seeds, Lean Meats, Grass-Fed Animals, Fish Oils, oils from fruits and nuts, etc.

Veganism:

This is more sort of movement and less of a diet. But I still consider this to have made such a huge impact that people think of this as a diet. In very simple terms vegans claim that we can source our food by not harming any animals in the process. The claim is that we could manage our eating habits just fine by using "vegan" alternatives that are mostly plant based and do not come from an animal. This is vegetarianism times a million. I categorise vegetarians in three different buckets.

Vegetarian: No meat, fish, eggs, everything else under the Sun.

Jain: Vegetarian but food that grow beneath the soil. This word is native to India.

Vegan: Vegetarian, not Jain but no animal involvement.

So yes, nothing from animals are allowed if you are vegan. Not even milk. Well, they do find different milks to satisfy their taste buds. I swear to God sometimes it's hilarious what vegans do. You see we cannot rewire our evolutionary habits and behaviours all of a sudden. But thanks to how it caught on, it's here to stay and will stick for generations. The first food man knew was meat. But we did evolve and due to tradition and culture, in the past thousands of years, we have vegetarianism arising. Vegetarianism is very popular. It has survived for so long, mostly due to religious reasons.

The biggest problem with the vegan diet is the sourcing and the macro problems. To produce vegan food, it requires a huge amount of processing. There is no food in the world that requires more factory work, chemical and biological processing than vegan food. More than meat and packaged food processing. And, they are highly, highly deficient in protein. Remember how much protein was important to us with respect to building muscle, losing fat, metabolism, etc?. Vegans have to literally scavenge for protein and even that is highly processed. Even if they get protein, it is not lean protein, it is higher protein but higher carbs as well. This can be exemplified by chickpeas and lentils that vegans use. Per 100g, they come with a big serving of carbs as well. I have learned enough than to argue with vegans. But, to each, his own.

Carnivore:

This, I can say, is the pure opposite of the vegan diet. This is also a movement more and a diet less, just like veganism. Vegans don't eat meat and everything is plant based. Carnivores don't eat plants and eat everything meat based. Yes, I had a laugh when I first came across this. It's almost like diet wars. This, also claims tons of benefits which again, becomes a field of study in its own.

Your Diet Given by Your Michaels/Gym Trainer/Coach:

This kind of a diet is a pure no go from my side. The majority of the world is okay with someone else preparing a diet and giving it to them. I completely oppose this idea for obvious reasons like - there being lack of empathy, lack of lifestyle alignment, no long term sustenance and many many more. It's ironic how people came to a position where you'd let others dictate your eating habits. It baffles me. Take advice, yes. Learn from folks, granted. But eat what they say when you live two different lives? I can't ever see a learned self doing that. Majority of these diets are not macro based at all. They are just a list of foods or meals that you should have and resemble more of a timetable. This is called the "diet chart".

Let me be honest, if you hand people a diet, most will not follow it, don't even ask me how many times I have passed to friends, family, acquaintances one of these plans and they have never followed it. Even if they did it, it wasn't to be for long as life caught up, things change and shit happens. At that point one would become helpless and would have to go back to this "diet giver" again. You almost have him on subscription. As I say - "We ain't got no time for that."

Intermittent Fasting:

It is astonishing that this is even correlated to a diet. And I am sad that I have to put this in this chapter for it to fit into context. Intermittent fasting is a way of eating, a pattern more so than a diet. Remember, a diet has something to do with macronutrients. Intermittent fasting does not care about your macros or even calories for that matter. It cares about *when* rather than *what*. Very simply put, this is a way of eating in which you have a window of time dedicated in your day for consuming your food, i.e, do all the eating and a window of time dedicated towards fasting. Yes, like not eating. At all.

To exemplify this;

Let's say I fast from 10 PM in the night (when I finish dinner) to 2 PM in the afternoon (when I have my first meal) everyday.

I cannot eat anything after 10 and before 2. I can have a lunch, a snack and a dinner or whatever in these said 8 hours that I have kept for consuming all my macros.

During the fast, I have nothing, absolutely nothing. Water is allowed. The objective is to not spike insulin levels during the fast, it is a pure and pure fast, no food. This means only a very few drinks can make the cut during the fast. Zero to almost zero calorie drinks like green tea, black coffee are the most prominent, with no sugar of course as we know how carbs metabolise. Body's response to sugar and anything that metabolises spikes insulin levels will break the fast. That is what is generally agreed. The major fasting splits are (Fasting window: Eating window) 14:10, 16:8, 18:6, 20:4 or more anything beyond this would be considered one meal a day or OMAD.

Is this sustainable? Probably not and I would clearly understand if this is something that you cannot do with your work/profession or lifestyle that you have going on. But I have somewhat made it sustainable for myself. I don't recall having breakfast even once in the last 4 years. I regularly fast 14-16 hours a day, every day, sometimes more.

Apart from these, you have the military diet, the raw food diet, the Kenyan diet (what are they eating over there?), and the other diets you saw in the zoo.

You have probably witnessed these headlines or statements:

"Follow the Paleo diet and you will lose weight". "Follow the ketogenic diet and you will lose weight". Get this straight. Nothing, nothing of the above is true if you are not in a calorie deficit. The weight formula does not lie.

But, irrespective of whatever diet it is;

All of them surround around one and only one thing: MACROS. Get that crystal clear. Question them, enquire into them and challenge them. There are a million and one diets that will be marketed to you and more are yet to come. A layman here like aunt Ruchi may say, "Hey, look at this new diet, it seems promising, my friend lost 5 kilos doing this." But you will know that the new diet made her friend go into a deficit and cut down on some unwanted macros.

Regardless of all of these, I contend that the best diet is a diet that you have made and you come up with. Something that you are comfortable following, something that need not be forced, something that is second nature to you, something that is long-term (but flexible to short-term changes), something that you feel like is not dieting at all but you know doing this gets you to your goal. You see what I did there, what you are doing is not dieting, it's building a relationship with food, it's creating a lifestyle, screw that it's building long term habits.

The purpose of giving you a blurb of the major diets is because this covers the gamut of the noise that is in the space. Only by knowing what people are doing could you become an expert at creating your diets. And this diet - your diet, also is centred around your goals, your life, your conditions.

We learnt about eating. We learnt about the major macro splits. We learnt about the macros. All you need to do, is apply them in accordance with your goals and your life. It's that simple. Easier said than done however.

How to create your own diet? The 3 steps to CYD (creating your diet)

Step 1: Know how many **calories** you should be eating - according to your goals.

Let us take Kiara's example which is simple weight loss.

Maintenance calories = 2000

Consumption = 1700 calories eating at a deficit of 300 calories a day. Manageable. (training deficit may be extra)

CALORIES = DONE.........1

Step 2: Figure out your favourable **macro split** - According to your goals and lifestyle.

Let us take Michael's example, he wants to maintain (no surplus or deficit)

Maintenance calories = 2400

Consumption = 2400

Macro split = 30%-50%-20%, in the PCF order. 720:1200:480 (calories) 300C 180P 50F (actually 53.33F) (approx in grams)

CALORIES = DONE, MACRO SPLIT = DONE............2

Step 3: Know what **foods to eat**: According to your goals and lifestyle.

Let us take Aunt Ruchi's example: She just wants to lose weight.

Maintenance calories = 1800

Consumption = 1400, eating at a deficit of 400 calories a day. (training deficit may be extra)

Macro split = 40%-40%-20%, in the PCF order. 560:560:280 (calories) 140C 140P 30F (31.1) (approx in grams)

Food: Recall the food chart. She will add Lots of lean meat and lean cuts like fish and chicken. Eggs and Paneer are also in the mix. Does away with sugar and other simple carbs as this carb count of 140 is something she is used to eat in one sitting, this is for a day. Keep some calories for alcohol as she likes her weekend wine. Well, that, or maybe she uses an app. But, at the end of day, she wouldn't have eaten a gram above 140C 140P 30F.

CALORIES = DONE, MACRO SPLIT = DONE, FOOD DONE............3

Step by Step:

Calories > Macro splits > Foods that Fit into the macro split.

This was just about these folks. Your answers to the three steps may differ. And therein lies "your own diet" Are you at this point equipped to completely come up with your diet? Let me break it to you. It does take work. But the reward is highly asymmetric.

Chalking out foods that fall into your macros, choosing a split, picking out and knowing what food is more rich in protein, what are rich in carbs and similarly fat, scheduling and planning and cooking. That is what it takes.

For most people, and I will reiterate this clearly again, macro splits and all macro counting is not at all that necessary. In fact, for the most part, you should just track your total calories and protein. That is way more than 99% of the world is doing. Natural flow of things will take you from there. Doing it, is what is must. Just be cautious about the other two macros and fill the rest of your daily calories with them.

You see why a diet that is sculpted by you helps? It helps because you did it, your ego will not let you give up in the worst-case scenario. You have accommodated all possible things so there's no one to blame. You are living it and cannot put this on anyone else. If it were given by a third person, there was a definite chance for obscurity but here it is definitely not the case. You stand the highest chance of success if it is your product. Your brainchild.

People go to different lengths to hit their macros. They do "meal preps" which is preparing your meals according to your macros 4-5 days in advance. People pay expensive subscription fees to get food delivered according to their macros. These are psychotic things from my dad's point of view. Frankly, I wouldn't disagree with him as I, having been there, felt only miserable. So what is the answer then? I did not write this book to tell you to follow the CYD, that's antithetical to the objective. But I had to mention it for you to get the lay of the land, how you'd approach your eating if you'd want to "scientifically" achieve your goals. It is not that hard. I don't want the world to suffer.

Creating your own diet is a wonderful short term strategy but it still becomes a time table. People will still fail because adherence is a huge problem. There are exciting foods, great parties, lovely events and beautiful things in the world. In this situation, even your diets that are coming from your own creative self will fail to stick. *"Why is this guy demotivating me?"*

Well, some will definitely follow it and find success. Some will be filtered out as they don't want to do the "hardwork". Some will be found wanting as they worked hard, did things but still were found guilty of breaking the flow too soon. What will you do then?

I hope that at this point you have come to the realisation that the term "diet" in itself is a nonsensical topic. You don't need diets, you need lifestyles, sure, when you want to cut down or get your body ready, we can optimise macros and cut back on certain foods and improvise training (exercise). But lifestyles and habits are what is needed. Something that takes no effort. To make such a simple point, I believe dragging you through the mud and chaos that is the dieting world (including creating your own diets) would be a risk worth taking. You did not become experts just by reading this chapter, you became equipped.

EXERCISE: One More Serving of Your Favourite Dish!

I want you to note down your top five favourite dishes your all-time top five. These dishes are you absolute FAVVVV!

Now, I want you to figure out how many calories including macros it has. Either split up the ingredients and add it on an app or if you're lucky and the item exists on the app, enter it. End result you know exactly the quantum calorie figures and macros.

I want you to tell this to yourself. "I can have it guilt free, I am smart" as many number of times as possible, out LOUD.

CHAPTER 8

BREAKFAST IS NOT THE MOST IMPORTANT MEAL OF THE DAY!

Breaking the dieting shackles, path to nutritional freedom!

***Scene: Me and Kiara in college. Working a whole day together for this fest.**

Kiara: Don't you want anything for breakfast?

Me: No, I'm good. Your sandwich seems nice though.

Kiara: Have a bite.

Me: No no. I don't eat in the mornings.

Kiara: WTH dude. I know you are on a diet, but you shouldn't starve.

------ Post lunch

Kiara: Is that a milkshake you're drinking? Whatever happened to the diet?

Me: Haha, someday I will tell you.

------ Dinner time

Me, to all the folks at college: I have some extra money from the collection, what say let's head out for drinks?

Everyone: Hell yes

Kiara: I'm in but I have to tell you one thing. Whatever diet you are on. I better hope its legal.

Me: One beer for you if it isn't.;)

Unlearning the World Famous "Breakfast" Myth:

If there's one thing that I would like you to take out from the book it would be the fact that breakfast is simply not the most important meal of the day. In fact, forget importance, it does not stand a place in my life and I believe shouldn't in many other folks' lives as well for reasons you will know soon. But again, I will not be suggesting that you tilt your life upside down because of one opinion. This book is written to help you do quite the opposite. Just being flexible goes a long way. But the fact remains the world's favouritism towards stuffing your body with carbohydrates (mostly sugar) first thing in the morning especially when these empty calories can be used for a filling lunch/dinner or a snack blows my mind. The morning bloat is really something one can avoid.

Imagine if I had a heavy lunch, some ice cream for snacks and also be able to save one doughnut for dinner. Would you think I was dieting? Hell no. Would you think that I was cutting fat and was on a very big deficit for weeks? And no, it wasn't my cheat day, (not such a lousy one of course). Everything I ate just "fits my macros".

The Concept of IIFYM:

My favourite form of "diet" is IIFYM or if it fits your macros. This term caught on pretty rapidly in the fitness circles. Following this means; to make sure at all costs that before you sleep, your macros are hit. You don't undereat or over eat any one specific macro. Let's assume that my macros are: 180P, 200C and 50F.

As long as I hit these, I am safe. When I wrap up my day, I need these macro numbers show up on my app, mind or notebook, wherever you're accounting them, to be as close as possible.

Maybe you would encounter a possibility of a bigger lunch today as you had a meeting with your business partner at a restaurant. Skip breakfast in that case, save calories for lunch. And no, your body won't starve if you skip a meal. Infact do it often. It helps. Maybe you went past your favourite ice cream shop that you loved as a kid. Go-ahead have it, I beeping insist, have that ice cream, no one's stopping you, you however get little carbs for the rest of the day and have to balance out the protein. You choose to have a 6 egg white only omelette for dinner for that very same reason. At home there is a doughnut that is sitting in the fridge left by your mother and it would get spoilt if it wasn't consumed by tonight. Alright, have it if you have enough carbs + fat (you know what foods have what macros only by counting them for a fair amount of time) left in your day but the dinner is equally balanced with lesser carbs and fat + filling out the protein that's left. And voila, there, you've dieted (infact pretty strictly) and no one, probably not even you would think that this was troublesome. You ate what you wanted, you did not stress out and you did not stick to a "diet chart". The macro math and the weight formula will not lie. As long as you are hitting them with whatever being your goal you are on track.

I and many would like to call it as **FDL - Flexible Dieting Lifestyle. (Note this, I will be usng the abbreviation commonly)**

Getting here is simply not easy. Even after going through so many processes and steps to get you to this point. You only have a major theoretical understanding, minor practical application. This only and only comes from real life practice.

You Will Not Be Doing This for Life:

The true nutritional freedom is achieved when you do not have to use an app or spend too much mental bandwidth on following a keto diet or a paleo diet or sticking to your macros. Simply as a result of education you must able to count what you most require, when the time is right and just be vigilant on all factors that influence your eating. Think about having a long the relationship that you have with food. And for that you need to completely understand food. Which you have as you have picked up this book and have come so far.

FDL is a beautiful thing. The most fittest people do it subconsciously but we are doing it with all the conscious till it becomes part of our subconscious.

A friend forces you for another drink, no problem, just cut down on the appetiser. You simply want another bite of that cake, don't fret, balance out your dinner. You don't want to be rude in front of company, no problem, balance out the rest of your day. Did you mess up on dinner or the last meal of the day? No problem, balance it out the next day so the sum of macros for the 2 day duration stays the same. (Do not stretch this beyond 2 days as it simply dominoes into entropy)

The best thing about this is it accommodates for everybody and everything and every possible situation. It is exhaustive. You can have Chinese, Italian, Indian, at will. You know to balance while others don't. You get to be on track, get fit while others keep munching. You can eat anything and everything until and unless it fits your overall calories and macros for the day.

A step ahead, intermittent fasting (IF) and fasting in general in my version of FDL:

The Marvel of Fasting:

Fasting, specifically, intermittent farting in a dieting context has tons of benefits. The main one being skipping breakfast or an extra meal that you simply do not need to eat.

We briefly touched upon the topic of intermittent fasting. Especially in FDL, Intermittent fasting is the mainstream adaptation of that which also has multiple benefits.

Listing down the benefits of fasting in general which is a divine habit that is simply amazing.

1. Aids fat loss. Not weight, fat. During your fasting period the body undergoes a lot of changes, for the work that you do, the body cannot use active glycogen as energy as you haven't consumed anything and sometimes for energy it does have to tap into the fat reserves. If you work out fasted, even better.

2. Helps make up for yesterday's mistakes. (Messed up your dinner, skip your breakfast, FAST, get back to zero).

3. Helps you eat bigger meals as you skip a meal or meals together. Mostly breakfast is thrown off.

4. Longer fasts (24-48 hours+) produce ketones, and you know what that does.

5. Reduces insulin resistance or to speak in layman terms, your dependency on glucose for energy. This = lower blood sugar levels and your sugar/sweet/carb cravings slowly wane.

6. Saves you money on the extra meal.

7. Allows for tastier meals as you can have little cheats here and there.

8. Accommodates any sort of life.

9. There are other proofs for things like improved mental clarity, concentration, repair of body tissues etc. I'll leave that up to your curiosity to learn. But as a general habit of wellbeing, fasting is clearly unmatched. Its mainstream adaptation is intermittent fasting, which is doable and really like a trick out of the bag if you master it.

Remember, getting to this level is a task. Takes weeks to months to almost years of practice to be able to fast for 14+ hours consistently. And beyond this one can even go to 20-24-36-72 hours fasting. Having done several long-term fasts, I can tell you that the changes are unbelievable both mentally and physically.

With all that said and done, the real challenge to fasting still lies in people not believing in it.

Society advising it as dangerous and unnatural. Not pushing through the initial pushback and fighting on. Folks like my dad who have not fasted for more than six hours their entire life feel like they're dying of starvation.

If you are making these changes in your body, especially when it comes to eating patterns after having gotten used to so many things right from the birth, the body is obviously going to give you pushback and withdrawal symptoms from your old habits. People will face mental and physical problems. But if you're fighting through it, rest assured you'll see the best out of life. This is not a gimmick. It has enough scientific backing. This fight, if won, can get you eat or drink anything you want. Such a feat obviously requires sacrifice. Believe me, when I eat that bite of pizza without giving a single "flying beep" I know that it has been worth it!

Fasting is a very big lever when it comes to this Flexible dieting lifestyle or FDL.

You simply do not know how much changes if you just choose the timing and not the content of your food. Read that again, timing of food, not content.

So yes, now I hope you understand why I hate breakfast. If you don't share the hate with me, it's alright, you can balance out the rest of the day by eating whatever you please as long as it fits your macros. You know, IIFYM. There are tons of places where I can allocate my carbohydrates (thinks about Indian ginger chai with milk my favourite). Why my version of FDL works is because it is a mixture of all these famous diets in one + fasting.

Did vegan for lunch. (Had a vegan cheesecake from this new bakery)

You probably did Paleo for a snack (Ate a fruit)

Did Keto for dinner (Steak + Avacado)

And so on.

Here is my word of caution however. Do not go overboard with FDL. If you say "Hey I'm going to balance it out" and do whatever you want, you will lose track and end up in a very bad position. This leads to what I call fitness entropy. Everything should have a purpose. Hard work can be thrown to trash if you are not holding yourself accountable. There is a method to this madness, do not forget. If you feel that you're slacking, stopped seeing progress or if your body is telling you (and it does) that something's getting too much, then, you are simply not hitting your macros. The weight formula doesn't lie.

This is nutrition in freedom. I cannot stress upon this enough. Getting here takes time, effort and real energy if you do it without having read anything up until now. But if you have read everything up until now and at least are on the way to work on internalising most things, you can expedite the process like no other.

All you have to do is practice, make changes, do iterations, adapt and build on this so that it fits your lifestyle and do not ever speak about dieting or diet charts or losing/gaining weight because of food ever again. Do not consider reading this means job done. I will reiterate what was said before in chapter 5, "You can't live on a diet, lifestyles are long term, in fact, habits and education is longer term". Getting here makes fitness a "Piece of cake" for you. Literally.

EXERCISE: Let's fast!

I want you to fast. I mean, I "suggest" that you do. Pick a day, have a light dinner early the previous night, fast for as long as you can. Regular fasters, you can 1.5x your previous longest fast. Mine is 54 hours so I shall try to one up it. If yours is 12, try 18, if it is 7 and you are a regular eater try 12 or 14 hours.

Do it this one for the sake of your picking up this book. It is completely your choice whether you choose to continue to do this on occasion or even regularly or not. But having done it once at least once gives you so much. Make a note of your experiences; mind, body and mood wise.

During the fast only water is allowed. No digestible food.

CHAPTER 9

PICK YOUR EXERCISE POISON

Scanning everything, cherry picking the one you want, taking it home!

Scene: Me and Michael at the gym

Michael: I am thinking of getting this fitness certification.

Me: Great.

Michael: This makes an expert on like 20+ training methods, I get to know a lot.

Me: That's wonderful man. Do let me in on some of the things you learn.

Michael: Once I get it, I'm going to make everyone who knows me shredded.

Me: Whoa, hold your horses. People have lives you know.

Michael: You should get one too.

Me: Haha no. That is great, I am open to learning more about it in the free time. But anything that I do, as a training activity, I try and bucket it into what I call "The Big 4". "Then I went on and gave him a gist about it).

I'm not an athlete, nor is this my profession. It's that way for 99% of this world. I do not want to learn the latest on what kinesiologists have come up with in conditioning or what new method popped up that created a buzz on social media. This way of think helps me get the job done without losing my sanity. I am open to education myself and experimenting for sure but I want to be free. It's just exercise. I have built a relationship with it.

Nutritional freedom is the freedom to eat anything whilst being grounded with respect to what your goals are and how your lifestyle is structured. Fitness freedom is the ability to look like how you want to.

Just like for nutritional freedom you do not require diet charts or diet or dietician or nutritionists. The same way, if you clearly understand more than the fundamentals of exercise and sharpen your knives with some key concepts, nobody can touch you. You will create plans on your own, improve and self-optimise.

Here is a thing that is tough about exercise over and above the fact that exercise in itself is tough for people. You really have to give it time. To get a hold of it, to master it or even start to actually enjoy it. Unlike food, which we optimise on a daily or weekly basis. Exercise is a longer game. I am speaking of years, decades and more. This has to be very clear in everybody's mind.

Here's a question. Are you a "I can exercise but can't diet" person or "I can diet and eat well but hate exercise" kind of a person? You see a majority of folks say that they are the former. But, if you know FDL, you will not fall in that bracket. You do not have a problem dieting.

I have seen very few fall in the latter category. It is easier to move your body than your mind. That is the only inference. Such a revealing one. However, just being exercise savvy will not get you far. By all means your workouts or form of chosen activity must be meaningful, controlled and last thing - with a sense of direction or heading towards a goal.

Without these 3, you will not last in the exercise game. It tends to last as long as a summer break for most. Creating a regular 5 or more days of working out habit, going to the gym, these things are really tough. Doing the workouts is never a problem. Soon enough you will enjoy it. Half of the battle is won by getting yourself to open the gym door or putting on the workout clothes. It is the very first step that matters. This game is won in the mind.

You have quite the grasp on some of the basics of exercise and activity. Until now training and exercise was synonymous to us. But, from now on;

Training: Your workout regime. Eg: Weightlifting, Cardio, Crossfit, Pilates, Spin etc

Exercise: One particular movement or form of movement. Eg: Bicep Curls/Squats/burpees

Your chosen form of training should depend on how you want to look long-term. This is a really important question. Everybody has a "type". What is your "type"?

Whenever you are doing any sort of training or working out, sneak in these questions in between, yes, bang in the middle of your workout, I want you to sincerely ask yourself these questions.

1. Is dream physique achievable this way?

2. What sort of body looks good on me? Does what I am doing help me in any which way? How so?

3. How do I want to look 10/20/30 years from now? How do I get there?

4. Can I see myself doing this 10/20/30 years from now? Do I genuinely like it?

5. Do I really know what I'm doing or am I just unmindfully doing what's told?

More often than not, people skip the basics, I did too, lost years in the process. Kiara's first ever fitness conversation with me ended this way - (she jumped straight to the main thing) What should your workout plan look like? "Monday through Sunday, rest days included, what should I do? Give it to me!"

Right answer? Well the answer I gave her is to never get herself into a situation that prompts her to ask such a question in the first place.

The approach to training is the same as food. Master your basics, build from scratch, put yourself in a position where you can build your own workout plans taking into account your goals and lifestyles and adhere to it. There is always room to learn more exercises, variations, add your own iterations. But, making or programming your own routine, like we did for FDL is the first step towards taking accountability and giving yourself a better chance at success. Once you get hold of it, you have your "fitness freedom". No guy/girl can tell you anything nor will you have to go to anyone for the most trivial of things. Like how Aunt Ruchi asks anybody with a half decent body this question - "What exercise do you do to reduce side fat?"

The Inside and the Outside:

For all practical purposes, from a physical fitness point of view, I look at body as 2 things: THE INTERNAL BODY and THE EXTERNAL BODY.

What's that?

Internal - Lungs and heart

External - Muscle, layer of fat and water

Again, I am talking purely from a "fitness" point of view. There is no need for a medical inference to be drawn here.

Well, if you recall, in chapter 6 we learnt about controlling muscles, fat and water. We also touched base upon what levers you can use to control or regulate them mostly but from an eating point of view. For most beginners, fat and water can take a back seat. For intermediaries and sane people, water takes a back seat. Only outlier situations and experiments allow for you to tamper your water composition. Too much water and too little water are both non optimal situations. Still a good weapon in the arsenal mind you. Muscle, however is the most important of the 3 if you did not realise already. You ought to know as much as possible about it. It almost feels like it is the answer to everything (I exaggerate).

From an exercise point of view, you cannot do much about fat and water over the short term, but you sure can do a lot about your heart/lungs and muscles. And, guess what the The Big 4 are directly related to this.

It is necessary that we learn about our muscular system, coupled with how our heart and lungs function due to the stimulus of exercise. Not as a student who is about to write a thesis on this biological topic but as a mindfully fit person who did not just "wing it". Muscle occupies so much space in our bodies, it's one of the pillars of our structure. It is connected to our metabolism, a determinant of our body composition. You would be a fool to overlook the strength of your own muscles. Stop reading, look at your body, take a clear look at how hard and big it is, how much of muscle can you really feel? Regardless of how much ever muscle you are packing, it is less. It is insanely valuable. Hard to get, easy to lose. Same goes for lungs and the heart, pivotal to your survival and a barometer to determine how fit you are.

Maintaining physical fitness means from a general common folk point of view - The well-being of 1) muscle 2) heart, 3) lungs. Things become so simple if you look at it that way. This way of thinking is no nonsense. And we have only a certain amount of years in which we can accumulate them and nurture them. Aging cannot be stopped, but if these 3 are managed, it can certainly be delayed. Yet, most people don't consider this when they talk about exercise. They go to the gym or hop on a cycle and just "get it over with". Knowing the physiological and biological effects of a certain stimulus or training method can really help us.

Bringing Back The Big 4:

Aerobic/Resistance/Balance and Flexibility.

Just like diets there are a million training methods propping up. But whatever they may be, largely they fall in 1 or more of these buckets. Michael does Crossfit Style training. On the face of it, a new age well rounded training method. But still, any exercise that he does, falls in one or more buckets of "The Big 4". That is how good the model is.

If it is not activating, effecting or bringing considerable change in your 1) muscle 2) heart or 3) lungs, stop it, it is not exercise/training, it is something else. Example here is walking for 100 meters to the grocery shop. "That ain't no exercise."

What happens when we train?

Effect of the 4 The Big 4 on Muscle:

Muscle can only be activated through resistance. So when you are training by providing force or building tension, you're effecting the muscle. It isn't a surprise that my favourite form of training is resistance training and I'd advise it to anybody walking the face of the Earth. Building, shaping and strengthening the muscles is under appreciated. We understood that protein is the building block of muscle from a food standpoint. But, from an exercise standpoint, they can only be activated by providing resistance exercises. And when provided with resistance, **it pains.**

All sorts of training, in some or the other way use and need muscle, but some work them more than others.

Effect of the The Big 4 on the lung-heart connection:

The heart and the lungs are involved in all sorts of training, again, some affect them, or work them better than others.

Most of your training activities, especially cardio (the name in itself is a giveaway) activities are possible because of the interrelationship between the heart and the lungs. Lungs take in oxygen and breathe out carbon dioxide. Oxygen is necessary for the heart to survive and pump blood all across the body. It is exactly what happens in your body whenever you do any sort of a workout. This in fact happens even when you are not doing any sort of a workout. But the rate at which these two function definitely changes when you are.

Whenever you are doing any sort of an exercise, you breathe at a higher rate as you need more oxygen, the heart as a result starts sending blood to all parts of the body, the muscles are used. The more this happens the more calories you burn. End of story. You can experience this for yourself when you run for a long distance - you feel breathless, or you crank out 25 push ups, your chest gets filled up a bit - "the pump". Indication that something "happened". When the heart and lungs are worked, you feel **"exhausted"**.

Intensity and training?

LISS Training:

Low intensity steady-state is LISS. The word itself says it. Majority of your aerobic, flexibility, strength exercises fall in this category. Low intensity steady-state cardio. Low Intensity steady state resistance training. Low intensity anything. Here, you are performing or exercising at a normal to medium of your maximum heart rate. Usually, this is the lesser than 70%. The heart rate differs from person to person. The benefit of this is that you can do it for long durations and burn more calories at ease. Because maximum intensity at all times is not sustainable, LISS is a go to and a part of anybody's arsenal when it comes to getting a good workout. LISS is often attributed to cardio only but I believe LISS is how most people exercise. Looking at phones, taking pictures, talking, etc while on cardio machines. Jogging, Running, Walking, Cycling, at ease weightlifting, all come under this category. Most training methods we know, even though they cause sweating for me are LISS.

HIIT Training:

High intensity interval training. As we have progressed, exercise has also evolved. HIIT, also most commonly attributed to cardio, is a game changer evolutionary find. We gleaned that training (aerobic exercise mainly) and its relationship between the heart and the lungs is pivotal when it comes to burning calories.

HIIT is a concept of training that makes the body do something called anaerobic respiration.

In this case, the body, cannot just of rely on the heart and lungs for energy. Anaerobic exercise asks of the body for more energy than aerobic exercise can give. For this, oxygen is not enough.

Simply put, this is LISS exercise on steroids. Metaphorically of course.

This takes shape when you do extremely intense exercise over short intervals of time. The intensity is so high that the body is forced to tap into glucose and stored fat in your body as energy. Both cardio and resistance training can be anaerobic. This is because it is completely dependent on the intensity of the workout and that can be figured out via heart rate.

It is generally considered, irrespective of whatever training you are doing, you will be in the anaerobic zone if you are upwards of 80% of your normal heart rate. And normal heart rate changes according to age and relative factors, google it. It is very difficult to sustain being in the anaerobic zone for a long duration but it is not stopping us from being in that zone for short intervals of time and taking the use of such form of exercise to burn more calories, activate muscles in a different sort of way. Nothing burns more calories and is easily effective in tapping into the stored body fat like HIIT. So, if you don't like doing long hours of cardio, do HIIT. Escape normalcy.

When do you know what training is affecting what?

Like everything, these models are my thought experiments. I devised this to know what really my workout consisted of. Whether I was concentrating on one thing or the other? Were my muscles or heart or lungs being worked? You know when your muscles are doing most of the work and you're feeling tremendous pain, a good pain (weightlifting) vs when you're panting for breath,i.e, lungs and heart doing most of the work. (long distance running)

Here is a rate card on how each of the top training methods fare when it comes to pain vs exhaustion.

Type of training	Pain/Exhaustion
Weightlifting/Traditional Gym	Pain
Crossfit	Both
Powerlifting	Pain
Calisthenics (Bodyweight Movements)	Both
Yoga	Neither (haha, no I am not kidding, power yoga is a bit different though)
Zumba/Any dance fitness	Exhaustion
Pilates	Both
Anything done HIIT Style	2x the pain/exhaustion and stars

Please recall: Aerobic training types burn more calories in one sitting. Eg: Cardio.

Resistance training burns more calories at rest, this is because your metabolism increases along with the increase in muscle mass. Eg: Weightlifting.

Exhaustion burns more calories, pain builds strength, which has a longer tail reward.

Some of the exercises contribute more towards building and managing the muscle while some towards activating the heart and lungs. Your cognizance of what you're doing matters a lot. You can practically draw this table for any sort of training/activity you come across. Based on this table, your lifestyle and your goals, you make the choice of what you want to do. Then your body is a result of consistently doing it, long term. This exactly mirrors the approach we took to dieting. Where we scanned the market for diets to get the lay of the land. Once we did so, we were more than capable of building our own systems and habits.

Flexibility and balance exercises usually take a back seat for beginners as they are more advanced iterations of activity as a whole. Things that your natural curiosity after reading this book will allow you to delve into. They are very important however when it comes to tackling the long-term game of exercise, when you span into years and decades. Some, argue that they should form the basis of all exercise and should take the front seat.

You should always mix it up. Long-term, your goal should get hooked to one or 2 things, so that you are motivated, playing within your circle of competence, while, in the short-term you should be open to experimenting and smoothening the edges. Eg: a professional bodybuilder with a bulky, boxy body. No judgement. Can do yoga to improve his stretchability. Nothing wrong, he maybe, wants to avoid injuries or got a free pass to try out a class. We know what his primary importance is. Conversely, a yoga instructor with a slender, yet flexible body (this is not a generalization) who has never lifted weights can definitely try it out to look more aesthetic, get stronger and "filled up". Muscle helps him do this. These are hypothetical examples. If you love something, for example - dance/zumba as your main then go for it, that is your "hook" to keep you fit. But do not become a one trick pony.

You will find yourself and many other people in these dilemma inducing scenarios. It's you, who always decides. Do something that you feel you **want** to do, that you **feel** will help you achieve your goals. Do something that you know for sure and can learn more of and can sustain long term. Do not again, be a one trick pony. Kiara finds her yoga time very helpful to relax. No problemo, the world is free. Go do it.

A fanatic Yogi or a Pilates girl would most probably not bat an eye when she hears anything remotely away from her specialty. It's her be all and end all. But as a reader of this book, please do not become that for your own good. Knowledge, ultimately helps. Experience and diversity will also help during times of need. I will take Michael and my examples here. If we just stuck to weightlifting at the gym and did not care about other ways of keeping ourselves fit, we would have both lost shape and gained a ton of weight doing during the coronavirus lockdown. **Hint:** We did not.

Now that we understand the gamut of what exercise can do; What is my pick? In fact, forget my pick, what is the world's pick?

With all said and done, weight or strength training has proven to be the most logical, replicable, easy and prolific way to get jacked. People love lifting weights, it is an addiction. Even for the odd one out who is not a "weights" guy or a girl. They just haven't ridden the wave for a long enough time yet.

Your microscope "hook" could be one thing (Like mine is weights) but you as an individual, you should be malleable and else you will plateau. This malleability helps you sustain this long term.

What if a person just does Yoga (and nothing else) and expects to lose 30 kilos? She ever gives her body a hint of intensity. They will never be able to see drastic weight loss results. Just one thing for her entire life with little to no knowledge of anything else reduces her chances of success.

Whatever the case, you should be doing activity, reepeatedly throughout weeks, months, years until it is second nature to you, part of your character. The goal should be to walk like a 40 year old man when you are 70. That's the main goal.

EXERCISE: Social Media Check!

How many right kind of people do you follow on social media?

I want you to go check your social media accounts. Clearly see how many people you follow provide you with Fitness/Health/Dieting/Self Care related content. I want you to question who these people are, what their background is are they genuine? As a thumb rule I want you to follow at least five well-known, **non-influencer type,** subject matter experts in the field.

These are scientists, PhDs, business owners/entrepreneurs in the field or even notable experts. But seriously, not run of the mill bloggers or influencers with a good aesthetic feed.

CHAPTER 10

GETTING YOU BACK TO THE GYM!

The 4 walls that give you freedom.

Scene: Me at aunt Ruchi's house. Again!

Me: Another Paratha please!

AR: Yes, coming. You will burn all of it in the gym right? You dirty fellow. I want to see you healthy like you were before. You're becoming scrawny by the day.

Me: Yeah, after this, I better be hitting the gym. This is my refeed day. I'm cutting.

AR: Everyday should be your refeed day. Anyway, Anushka (her daughter) goes to this dance class everyday, her friends seem to lose weight but she does not. Do you think she should join the gym for better results? Like You? Who's your trainer there?

Me: For god's sake aunty she is 12, let her be. Also, 1 last paratha. Please.

AR: Okay. But I don't want her to become like me. I'll put her into any coaching class but I don't want her to face my arthritis problems when she gets old.

Why do you see more gyms than Pilates studios?

Why do you think weights, barbells and dumbbells sell more than yoga mats?

What makes treadmills and stationary cycles part of every big home that has enough space for equipment?

Everybody has a fitness hook, I have made it clear that mine is the weights. No fancy stuff. The tried and tested neighbourhood gym. With so many ways and methods of quick fix, FAD solutions coming your way, why does the GYM remain undefeated?

Its right in your neighbourhood, well for some, it's at your home!

If you look back in time, tracing the approach that our ancestors took towards training, you would realise that we have come a long way. What we see in practice today and the colloquial understanding of the word "workout" is an improvisation of what was done hundreds and thousands of years ago. On the face of it, it sounds as if we are doing something way different than what our ancestors did. But we frankly are not, we have shrunk that part of our lives rather. I contend that fundamentally, humans, irrespective of whatever gibberish sort of workout arises on the corner, have only a few physical capabilities and as a corollary, have not progressed any much better than what the greeks for example used to do. Sure, we know more science, we have better records, we know more about the world, we can use tools and levers but what we can do has in fact minimised. Think about it, Pheidippides ran the first marathon barefoot in those ages, people went to wars frequently, hand built amazing monuments, nobody obese in sight. Fitness was not a lifestyle choice, but a civic duty. Pick up some time and read about physical fitness in the Ancient Greek Era. You will be left flabbergasted. We have become intelligent but our outer physical self has become inferior.

In the 21st century, we are finding the easy, efficient way out, "technology will help us workout better". Technology will help us do a million things for the better of our life, granted. But I still am a contrarian when it comes to technology having a sustainable, scalable, impact on humans having a solid outer, physical body. Nature is the answer to that. Can we go outside and lift rocks, logs and run on stones like centuries past? No. Whatever you say, even with all the innovation in the field, I still do not believe we have progressed much from the good old gym. The good old gym, for me, is the pinnacle. The answer to most fitness questions. Not martial arts training or Pilates or Zumba, but the weights, the bars and the atmosphere of a dedicated time to improve the body is the closest we can get to what the greeks did. And my god the greeks did wonders.

That is the reason why people refer to the term "Body like a greek god". Aesthetic, beautiful and a treat to the eyes.

The gym is most synonymous with bodybuilders. Yes, those who go perform at those bodybuilding shows. Although a majority of them are fake, steroid infused shitshow, there is a lot to learn from bodybuilders, their world and their life. Their circle of competence is the outer human body, its appearance. They know more than any person on this topic. Sometimes more than researchers thanks to first hand experience. This is both good and bad, but let's focus on the good. It's not a matter of chance or coincidence that the first thing that comes to people's minds when they think of a workout is the good old gym. This is called "Strength training" and often involves the art of weight lifting. It is because of centuries, decades, years of us doing so many things, did we find an efficient and effective way of training.

Strength training is a part of the Resistance bucket of The Big 4.

There is a whole field of study on this, a mine that does not stop producing. For us to get to our objective, a small dive into this topic will undeniably help us.

Training for Strength

We learned so much about the muscle and how it can be activated through resistance and resistance only. The traditional art of lifting weights has evolved for years and has given us a perfect opportunity to be able to provide muscle with great tension or resistance. Strength training is the best known lever to control muscles. It is a level above just normal resistance work which can be done by examples like Pilates, Calisthenics, bodyweight movements and the like. Strength training or often considered traditional weightlifting in the gym is the best bet we have to manage muscle. At will. There is so much one can learn by just taking an aerial view of a bodybuilder's life.

The constant contraction and relaxation that happens during a weightlifting session or any strength training session for that matter is what enables the muscles to break down and then grow. And nothing aids muscle than a bit of weight. Heavy weight. I cannot stress enough, the understanding of this concept can spiral your results at the gym.

Strength Training as an Alternative to Spot Reduction:

People who regularly do strength training, As opposed to any other format, do not appear "fat". I do not mind telling this "n" number of times. Spot reduction of fat is a no go, i.e, you cannot choose where you can lose fat from. But, your entire body is covered by muscles. Muscle dominates your appearance. Adding muscle to the place where you, by nature, pack a lot of fat (abdominal area for most, face for some and chest for others) can give the area a whole different look. This is the miracle of muscle. You can make it look like there isn't necessarily that much amount of fat just with the presence of muscle that is so dominating.

So, if you want to get the dream physique, if you want to be "toned", or plain and simple if you want to be fit. You better get to lifting weights.

Muscle Protein Synthesis and Breakdown:

When you're doing any sort of resistance training, you are breaking muscle down, not building it. This is not for you to become an expert at muscle science by any means, but, while strength training, or doing any strength training exercise, the body breaks into the muscle fibres creating tears and damage. This amount of damage depends upon the stimulus. More the stimulus, more the damage. (Compare weightlifting stimulus vs Pilates stimulus) It is after this stimulus does the muscle "recover". There is a window of time upto 2 days right after this workout, that enables the body to build back up, i.e, get ready. Compare this to how your body heals after it bleeds from a cat scratch. Protein as we know is the best way to help build it. That is why people drink protein shakes after workout Think about the protein muscle connection again. See, it all makes sense now. This process of muscle protein synthesis is what helps muscle grow. It may be counterintuitive but more the damage, more the synthesis.

Why are we talking about muscles so much? This is because I do not want you to be the average person who goes to the gym. You can't learn on the job. It is not harmful to equip yourself.

To increase the damage, you can add things like volume (no. of exercises and reps), quantum of weight, length of training, etc. Easily put, harder the workout, better the chance at muscle growth. As you keep stimulating your body through weights, your body keeps getting used to it and your rate of synthesis will not be the same. This happens when you add months, years and decades to your training. The process of building the strength and size of the muscle is called muscle hypertrophy.

Read the next lines carefully. When you are not stimulating your body enough through resistance, and are almost sedentary, the body undergoes the opposite of hypertrophy which technically is called muscular atrophy. This happens as your body instead of synthesising new muscles, it is breaking itself up. In essence, your inactivity can lead you to altering your body composition, instead of a muscular person that you once were, because of throwing diet and mostly training out of the window, your body fills itself up with water and fat. Increasing your body fat%. This is what happens when you suddenly leave the gym or stop working out.

Atrophy can also happen during times of extreme starvation, deep calorie restriction and other medical/biological reasons too but that is for another day. If you are not stimulating the muscles enough with the required protein and resistance, the body is forced to eat its own muscle for energy, to put it simply. This can also be called as Muscle Protein Breakdown. The amount of muscle in your body depends on the stimulus (protein, strength training, our 2 muscle levers). Because it cannot be stimulated all the time, it is easier to lose it than gaining it.

There is a reason why in chapter 6, I mocked the concept by saying - "Muscle is built when muscle protein synthesis is greater than the rate of muscle protein breakdown"

Okay, I promise you no more strength training jargon. That is left for the intellectuals and pros in the field.

The weight formula like always, applies. To add any amount of weight, even in this case, you need to be in a calorie surplus. But, beginners indulging in strength training have an unfair advantage. I used mine and I want all of you not to miss out on the chance.

It is a known fact in the fitness circles that new gym goers and new lifters go through a version of beginner's luck. Imagine you are new to the gym, you are not used to the stimulus priorly, you tend to see quick results. This is usually called as newbie gains. People gain a real good amount of muscle pretty quick when they are new to weights. This is a gold mine. Go fetch it, especially if you are young. That is why people see tons of results in their first year or so and things plateau. The beginning phase is the only phase where you can lose some weight and build some considerable muscle, yes almost and the only case of going against the weight formula. And no, it's not fat converting into muscle - it doesn't work like that. The only catch is that the beginning phase or the newbie phase takes some time to start producing results. A few months of genuine work is required. Some folks try so hard, almost make it to see the results and let go or stop just before the D day. They frequent the gym for 3-4 months and give up just when the time is ripe.

Strength Training is Broadly Done with 2 TOOLS:

1. **Machine or equipment assisted:** These are the machines/ equipment that are present in most gyms. Easy to do, tons of these, instructions given and most importantly does the job.

2. **Free weights:** These are the usage of non static machines. Free weights generally mean the usage of barbells, dumbbells and the like. I believe these to be one of the best inventions known to man. I exaggerate of course (or do I). These are your literal and not metaphorical levers for you to determine how you want to look. This topic in itself is a Galaxy of things to learn.

Strength Can Broadly Be Classified into 2 Types of Exercise Buckets:

a) **Isolated Exercises:** Targets and works mainly one muscle, assisted by max 1-2 secondary muscles.

Eg: Bicep curls (Main muscle - Bicep, forearms also used)

b) **Compound Exercises:** Targets and works 2-3 muscles, assisted by more than 1-2 muscles

Eg: Squats (Main Muscle - Thighs/Hamstrings/Lower back, calves, upper body muscles also used)

Exercises Can Be Learned:

This is by no means a workout book or an exercise book. There are at least 10 well-known exercises for each of the muscles in your body. And all these have their own variations. As you learn and do and explore your will for sure figure out more ways to activate them. Activation is key, not the exercise. So understand, internalise and concentrate on the basics. You can learn tons of exercises everywhere from the Internet to professionals to experienced lifters to innovators in the field. Some, you may just invent. Just learning exercises without understanding its function or vice versa is what leads to people not seeing results.

All You Need to Know Is 2 Things:

1) **What happens in the mind:** This cognisance, mindfulness of what muscle or part of the muscle you are planning on activating, working out, providing resistance for. Doing this helps create a mind - muscle connection that is a force of nature whenever you exercise.

2) **What happens outside:** The correct way, range of motion and posture of doing the said exercise.

All of this boils down to practice, ability to read up and learn about movements within exercises (eg: bench presses), willingness to take the tougher approach of mastering the theory and then putting into practice rather than doing exercises and then after some time spent doing it, realising its actual purpose and use.

Each muscle group may have multiple muscles, these can then have different areas, each area can be activated through an umpteen amount of exercises, some you may find already popular, some maybe that you learned as a result of tons of work. But that's your homework.

Strength training in the good old gym is accessible, learnable, teachable and everything easy. It should take up a majority of your gym time. It is, simply, a glaring answer to so many simple and complicated lifestyle problems we have. Just go, lift weights. Just go to the gym.

The gym is the body's mecca. Unlike other training methods, it is insanely flexible. It lets you do almost whatever and has no bounds. Having said that, like every topic. Establishing and setting your mind up with the basics goes a long way.

My Commandments of Programming Your Gym Time:

1. Quality Over Quantity.

Just doing the exercise as somebody teaches you to do it is not going to do the job.

a) Tension: The strain or the tension in the muscle is what determines it's activation. And the longer and stronger tension, the better it is for the muscle. Time under tension (TUT) is key for the muscle, not the half arsed repetitions. You can increase TUT either by increasing the weight/resistance, or by increasing the range of motion, or by increasing the time itself of the muscle under tension. So, if you just keep cranking out hundreds of repetitions of any exercise you have in mind, you lose the chance of being more efficient like you are doing the exercise.

b) ROM: Range of motion is knowing where the exercise starts, where it ends. It is the learning about the motion you are performing, and being mindful about it and doing it completely. You can do two reps with complete ROM, TUT and it would still not be equal to 8-10 reps with mindless effort and doing it to achieve the number. "My trainer told me 12 reps, so I did 12 reps" No. You did not. That should be the answer to any of your questions regarding how many reps I should do. It boils down to tension, it boils down to ROM.

c) Posture or Form: Posture and body positioning (form) are determinants of how well your exercise is done. Wrong posture would mean you are not activating the intended muscle or on the other hand, could lead to injuries. If you don't learn the posture of the exercise, you better not do it. Take time to master the form. Do it the right way, the intended way. A general rule is this, you do not sacrifice form for ease of doing or pleasure of lifting heavy. Simple.

So, the next time you come across any exercise, question these 3 things: How tension is applied, what is the range of motion and what is the correct posture to do it.

2. Concept of Splits

Do not do just one single thing everyday and expect results. Splits are hugely beneficial for a balanced looking body and surely keep you mentally hooked by mixing things up.

a) Muscle Splitting:

The bro split is a common term used for exercising one muscle group every day, usually performing various exercises of this muscle group, hitting a majority of them and that only becomes the workout for the day. Every day is for a designated body part in other words. Like Monday is "International Chest Day"

Just like how the bro split had a one muscle group a day approach. As we move towards being an intermediate lifter, to provide the body with the same amount of stimulus would not be called at progressive. Otherwise, results stop and one would plateau. Working more muscles, intensifying and diversifying the workout becomes necessary.

Advanced programmers of workouts usually include 2 to 3 muscle groups worked per day. Some even include the innovative concepts of push and pull split. Doing pushing exercises on one day and pulling exercises on another day keeping a separate day for legs. Some also mix it up, they incorporate the concept of the bro split/push pull/multiple muscles so as to fit into their goals. See here, flexibility.

Adding Compound Movements:

After learning that intensity and activation is necessary for growth or wellbeing of the muscle, people start finding cheat codes to achieve this. An answer to this could be steroids but the other answer is as close to steroids as possible. These are your compound movements. Yes, the exact movements/exercises that hit more than 2 to 3 muscles. Ancient Greeks always vouched for this. Doing this has significantly proven to burn more calories, increased activation and use of muscle, and also help in its growth and upkeep like no other. I mean everybody loves more muscle right? More muscle equals more metabolism equals more strength equals better body structure and so on and so forth. Hence, do not let go of your compound exercises.

b) Cardio and Extras Splitting:

Similar to how you split your muscles across the week, the other part of an essential workout is training the lungs and heart. For bodybuilders, this is through old school cardio. Usually through machines like treadmill, elliptical and cycling.

The allocation of your cardio could be split by days, by machines or any other way you choose it. The objective is to hit your deficit that you want to create in energy by burning the calories off. You can also split any other part of your routine this way. Maybe you like to swim for cardio or love to do jump rope, split this also across the week.

Whether you do cardio first or weight training first does not matter. Although weight training is done first as you have more energy in the beginning of the workout, some prefer it otherwise and it is perfectly alright. Kiara Hates cardio. So, she ticks that box first as she enters the gym and her mental load comes down.

3.   Are you a +/- or =

We don't want to work out for the sake of working out. No goals means no control over effort, as a result, no control over results. At any given point, a traditional "gym bro" is either progressive, regressive or staying put trying to balance it out. Knowingly or not, it is such a brilliant hook for you to keep at it. That is why I love the gym. It is always a + or a - or an =. Doing any 2 things at the same time leads to what I call fitness entropy again, doing work, but with no direction. We can learn a lesson from the bodybuilding world here. It is a very popular concept when zoomed out and looked at, gives us not only valuable info but key insights to manage our fitness lives better.

Bulking/Cutting/Maintaining:

Some professionals and intermediaries do these things called and bulking and cutting. In essence this is to change your body composition over the short term which in turn changes the looks over the medium-long term. This may not be something that common folk would want to do or endure, but just knowing the process is such a fitness lesson. For bodybuilders, this is bread and butter.

Bulking involves building of muscle mass which means being on a very good caloric surplus with higher protein of course. It is ridiculously tough and inconvenient to gain "just muscle" on the road of eating more. Just gaining muscle would involve just eating insane protein in a surplus calorie intake. That is practically impossible. Carbs help you get easy calories in and provides a free flow of easy energy which is very important in this bulking process. Hence, this surplus does bring in with it, some fat gain also. (remember; weight = muscle + fat + water for the most part).

Calorie surplus plus incredible strength training equals bulking up/becoming bigger. Bulking gets you big and thick. Do not confuse bulked up to fat or overweight.

Fact: *Research shows a maximum of 2 lbs or just under 1 kg of muscle per month is the most that can be gained naturally. This is with super focused training and rigorous optimisation of protein* *intake eating at (approximately in a range) 2 grams of protein per kilo of bodyweight or 1 gram of protein per lb of bodyweight. Put that into perspective - if you are 100 kilos or 220 pounds, you need to be eating 220 grams of protein in a day. That is way more than the average person's protein intake and is really tough to follow for months on end. Where that comes from, how many calories it is, you already know it and I am not helping you this time.*

So, we can say without a doubt that just lifting weights will not make you bulky as it is not that easy. Do not be afraid of lifting weights. You will just build a stronger "muscle you" hidden under the "real you" separated by skin. This makes you look structured, "toned" and aesthetic.

Cutting on the other hand is the exact opposite. In essence it is to retain as much muscle mass as possible and get rid of as much fat as required. It's like a sculptor's job. Just like how you just simply cannot just gain muscle mass, here you simply cannot just lose fat, along with the fat, you will lose some of the size (muscle) as you are in a calorie deficit. But the art is in minimising the very same. So how does one be in a calorie deficit and just lose fat? Well, just losing fat is not an option, you will lose muscle in some or the other form, if you are not on some steroids. Cutting does involve a lot of cardio along with strength training as a main pillar. Our primary goal is not one but 2 things - fat loss + muscle maintenance.

Because of the intensive relation between protein and muscle, a higher protein diet is another huge lever during your cutting phase.

So, caloric deficit plus incredible strength training plus vigorous cardio to get rid of unwanted weight (most of which being fat) is called cutting. Cutting gets you to look shredded/ripped and get those abs/vascularity and leanness to pop out. There are obviously more nuances to this but our understanding of the fundamentals of the cutting and bulking world helps us navigate our individual journeys way better. I have seen and so have you, many transformations, fat to fit revelations of people who already packed a huge amount of muscle mass, had a history of training, just cutting off the fat and revealing the shredded look. It is completely different from an obese or extremely overweight person's fat to fit transformation.

Summing up bulks and cuts. Why did I even bring this up?

You cannot bulk and cut at the same time because you cannot be in a caloric surplus and a caloric deficit at the same time. It's mutually exclusive. And, you cannot reach a position of "maintaining" until you have reached your goal body composition in the first place.

In fact maintaining is the goal for all of us. But it's elusive. Nobody can last a maintenance phase for long. No one wants to be married to the gym. Trust me, NO ONE. You need breathing room for other things in life. Eventually, people will have slip ups, life will get in the way. It 100% will and you'll have to self optimise to a + (bulk) or a - (cut) depending on how you want to look. Every "I'm just maintaining" endeavour leads back to a +/- scenario. It just does. Things don't stay the same for long. Does that mean you're not allowed to maintain? Heck no, as I told the goal is to get to be able to maintain. That is your freedom for the work you put in. I'd call reaching the level of being able to "maintain" is your FDL of training. You can name it FTL, Flexible Training lifestyle if you want. This was another thought experiment of mine that worked in reality. You have more or less your dream physique, who is to stop you? Keep the majority of the workouts the same and go try anything else under the sun. No other thing other than results you get from the gym, give you this freedom. If you don't immediately self optimise your external physical self in case of a slip up with a + or a -, it becomes a slippery slope and, in a few years, then you are on the road to what Aunt Ruchi, My dad faced. The gym lets you do the +/-,not in most other training methods. Sure, you get better, you improve and learn new things. But nothing gives you the flexibility of a regular gym. That was my intention to bring in the concept of +/-/=.

I myself, post losing the weight, looked like an amoeba. No shape, no muscle and no definition. I wilfully bulked up, built some muscle, did the dirty work and cut down on purpose diligently. Could I do it with just outdoor bodyweight workouts, yoga? Would I build considerable muscle? Heck No. The main work of losing weight can be done by many and pretty easily as you garnered early on with the weight formula. Smoothening the edges, going a step forward is what a very few do. Having done multiple attempts at bulking and cutting, I can tell you that there are lots of nuances in this but the more you are immersed in building on this concept, the more you will learn about controlling how you look. I believe knowing the concept of +/- and = is the key to having any control and accountability.

So, whenever you are programming, devising or planning a workout or training schedule or even thinking about it. Take these 3 points as bases:

1) Are you prioritising quantity or quality?

2) Are you splitting your work? Or are you blinkered and just doing 1 thing.

3) Are you aiming at a +/- or a =?

The gym goers, people who swear by strength training as their hook have a luxury. They have options. They are not constrained. Most of all, it works. Almost every other FAD training method resembles a cult. Almost an irreverence if you indulge in any other training method. When it comes to training, you cannot just blindly follow what has been running in the market.

Having the gym as your hook is great. Gym = FTL.

Why is this FTL great?

Muscle imbalances are common. For example, Kiara's right shoulder is more developed than her left. It's pretty clear. For that, you may need to work one muscle, here shoulder for the whole extra day. (Bro split)

Michael may be working late because of a project at work this month and can only work out three times a week, he/she can add in more muscles (push pull/2-3 muscles)

My dad may just have a single day in the week to work out, he may not even be able to go out of his apartment complex on this day. (just compound movements at the gym + treadmill)

Worst case, you want to do yoga, Gym has space.

You want to dance, Gym has space.

You want to run, Gym has the treadmill.

Just GO TO THE GYM.

You see, in normal daily life, you cannot expect to follow the constructs of the fitness society. I suggest you to question all these constructs that exist. Self programming your workout routine is the end goal. The folks who are at that level are the ones that you should be aiming to become. The gym approach with strength training is so easy and efficient that it gives you the flexibility. The other sects of training, not so much. Flexibility really works. This is long term sustainable.

Aim for freedom. Do not be bound. Be systematic, learn what needs to be learnt but be free. Freedom can only be achieved if you know enough, try enough. Freedom has a huge platform of knowledge. Just doing what you wish is also freedom but that is ignorant, most likely won't fetch you any result. This mindset will help you like no other. Let us not forget our main objective, the goal is not to remain in a constant state of Bulk +, cut - or maintenance. The goal is to know enough so that when life hits you, you know how to bounce back.

Often, people remember the tools and methods of building and shaping the body. What they often forget is the pillar concepts of what makes the body eat, why we eat, what makes us train, where we inherit certain concepts from, what helps us make better fitness decisions in general. Over one glean, a careful understanding of the pillars of their field teaches us, the common folk, so many things,

I really wish that you lift as much weight as possible, and make strength training a part of your routine. I hope everyone of you has a body like a Greek God. But, if that does not fit into your "reality", make use of what you have learnt as an investment in your fitness life. Irrespective of whoever you are, that should be the takeaway from the chapter.

EXERCISE: More of Them Muscles!

From head to toe, try and feel every muscle that you have. You don't need to know the name of the muscle but you just need to know that it exists. Wherever you feel flesh, identify it. Give each of these muscles a google search query name.

For example, you might come up with: Muscle that connects neck and shoulder at the back. (google tells you that this is Trapezius or traps)

Another example, you might come up with: Muscle that is on top of my thigh (google tells you its Quadriceps or Quads)

Then,

Google - how to activate.........(the said) muscle(s)

Do this for as many muscles you are curious about.

The rest is a mystery and a gift that I simply did not have enough words to put into this book. Just know that we are filled with muscles and our muscular body needs working on to look GOOD.

CHAPTER 11

A MENTAL BATTLE!

How to win the Psychological Game first? My top 15 tips.

By more means than one - fitness is a psychological game. Just maintaining and altering body composition in itself is daunting, tedious, scrupulous, energy consuming. Imagine the plight of people who have a lot of weight to lose or in the odd case, some weight to gain.

These are deep rooted physiological, biological, behavioural changes that you are asking from yourself. Literature, theories help, practice is what is needed. But it's clearly easier said than done. One can easily lose hope, motivation and multiple other stimulants even while practically applying theories, tricks and tips.

Hence, it makes sense for you to highly internalise the goals and find a really good reason for you to do it. Because, millions of people give up, hundreds of thousands of people just gave up today. Many just don't overcome the pushbacks.

The reward is too good for you to not push through those obstacles. Take it from me and a million others who made it to this side.

My Personal, Top 15 Tips. All Things "Mind" Related.

1.   Motivation vs Habits:

When it comes to fitness, motivation will definitely help, but if you depend on motivation or little spurts of pushing from your friends, family, yourself or anyone or anything for that matter, it will likely wane off. I remember a time when I used to watch one video of "workout motivation" on YouTube before hitting the gym after coming back from University. This worked for 5 to 6 weeks where that video view adrenaline would get me up and running, ready to grind it out. Slowly this waned off as well. Then I started cold showers. A cold shower before the gym to get every single inch of your body awake. Then I started looking at my old photos, looking at the progress that I had made. This too, helped for a while but it stopped quick and did not give me the push. I was like bleh, "I don't feel it today". There will be a million other versions of this "I don't feel it".

My story aside, I constantly see people finding sources of motivation in the form of alarms, music, timetables, checklist, resolutions, showers etc to get their ass to the gym. There is nothing wrong in doing this but please realise that you have to move past this stage when you are all excited and want to get motivated to the next stage of making it a habit. It is almost like brute forcing it. It doesn't matter that you forced it but you will be glad that you did.

Habits help you out long-term. Crank it out, do it, go to the gym in fact when you least feel like it. What if your general lifestyle required you to be at the gym one hour a day five days a week irrespective of whatever came? What if like your morning coffee or tea, working out is a part of life without any argument or questions raised? What if you had to work out like you took a dump every day?

I cannot stress this enough, do not seek motivation (and expect long-term results), do not look for gimmicks (and expect long-term results), make it a habit.

2. Battling Insecurity:

When we speak about the concept of insecurity, it usually has to do with the internal self and not much the physical external body. Should you be insecure if you are fat? Yes, you better be. Do not embrace "your curves" if you have not given it a proper go yet. Lots of people walk around being insecure about something that they have control upon. Sure, we cannot change your genetic looks, height, facial asymmetry and the like, but we can do a hell of a lot otherwise.

At any given point, if you are ever insecure about your body, first you need to get to an understanding that you can change it. The power is vested in you. Second, you need to understand that you cannot have the goal of replicating something or comparing yourself with somebody. Everybody is guilty of doing this, consciously or otherwise.

Read the next few sentences very carefully.

Here is my little rant on this topic post being a victim of it myself. *"You do not know their story, you do not know their genetic background, you do not know their experience, you do not know their authenticity, you do not know their journey, you do not know their upbringing, you do not know their forces, you simply do not know enough."*

You cannot in the right mind, with the billions of people that we have in population and multiple combinations that exist in the world, ever put yourself through the trauma of comparing your body to another human being. I am not saying it would be easy but it is second nature to us to want those big arms like the bouncer, dream of those abs like that actor, dream of those jawlines of the guy at the bar, etc.

Don't look at your external physical self, the body, as something that is easily replicable. There are multiple things that are deep-rooted in our genetics, DNA that we cannot alter. Some people are born with a good face structure, some are born with naturally well developed abdominal muscles, some are born with dimples, some have naturally broad shoulders, big arms, long face et cetera.

Insecurity, at least with respect to the body where I have some subject matter knowledge, will kill you, pretty slowly. This comes from a person who has lost more than half of his body weight today. My body is covered with loose skin and stretchmarks. Trust me when I say that these are true learnings.

Never be insecure, devise your ways to work around it. But, at the same time, it pisses me off to see people just throw in the hat and give up. "I can't do this, I will just be fat/unfit. Anyway, you can't change anything" These people are doomed. Eg: Aunt Ruchi, turning 39 soon, spoke about Kashmiri's and how aesthetic their faces and bodies are and how she will probably never get "there" irrespective of her diet. Kashmiris, through no fault or plan or of their own, but due to geographic, genetic and a thousand other reasons are the way they are. But here stands a woman in Bangalore, India, dreaming to become like them. Insanity.

My suggestion would be to maintain that fine line of balance of being envious/jealous just enough to motivate yourself and get that energy kicked in to try harder but not to the point where you sulk in self pity.

3.   Overeating Generation:

The first thing I want you to note as a 21st century human being is that you don't need to eat that much. This has to be one of the main takeaways out of this book. Our calorie intake has significantly risen. Even the poverty of today eats much more than the poverty of the old years. (No I don't mean food is bad). We didn't progress evolutionarily eating unwanted snacks emotionally filling our mouths crying, binging. Believe it or not our average calorie consumption per day in the 1960s was around 2500, as of 2018 it was 3600. That is a significant jump, and that stat brings in as you know weight gain, structural changes, body composition changes, obesity and yes fatter bodies. Compare your hunger to a beggar's hunger. Do you feel hungry every four hours/five hours? You see, the beggar does not. You will never see a fat beggar. Over a long duration your body's definition of hunger changes. And it all starts in the mind. So no, you are not "starving" at 7 PM cause you had an early lunch. Do not ever misuse the word "starve".

4.   The concept of Plateauing:

Plateauing is a general concept in science. Consider your fitness results on the y-axis of a 2 plane graph. Consider time on the x Axis. If you keep doing the same thing over and over again, i.e, effort being static, over a certain time, your graph will look like a plateau, flattening if you will. Without being progressive (moving upwards in the graph), without moving up the levels, testing yourself harder, doing more, your results will, by all means, plateau.

Use levers, concepts, underlying foundations that you have learnt about food and fitness in general from this book, break through those plateaus. In a long enough time-range, everybody plateaus in one or the other things but the key is winning the battle against the little plateaus.

Weight Loss Plateau:

Perhaps the most important and widely known plateau would be the "weight loss plateau"

If over a short duration you are doing everything right and you are still not seeing results then that should not be a cause for concern. As long as the macro math, weight formula, The Big 4 and related concepts that you have applied is right, you will be seeing results and your life will be changing. But there's a chance that after seeing an initial spurt of good results, you suddenly stopped seeing it. This most commonly happens during weight loss. It is a clear case that weight loss is not a linear progress. It will have its ups and downs. Some variables in your life are just beyond control.

If you were ever in a plateau i.e. lost some kilos then it "became tough" "results stopped" (you plateaued) so you ended up actually giving up like millions, remember, this thing has its ups and downs. You have to try harder. It gets tougher as you go before it gets easy and you've got to push through and dig in. You have to try the tips and tricks that you've learnt and you have to go back to the basics. It's true when they say that doing the same thing over and over and expecting different results is stupidity. You might wake up a kilo or two heavy one day just out of nowhere after doing possibly everything right and you would not even know about why it happened or be able to reason it. Break those plateaus. Everybody has them.

5. Letting Loose. Learning from Popular Culture and Alcoholism.

Everyone likes to have a good time. Let loose. Have fun. Let me give you some good news, you do not need to sacrifice life's pleasures or vices for your fitness. At least after having read this book. One such vice would be alcohol. For some it might be a good old cigar. For others it might be raving and partying their faces off. Doomed are those who think balancing all aspects of life is not possible. Sure, do not go overboard, damage your internal organs and overall health as that would be general advice to any human being. But abstinence or restriction is something I would not suggest unless you really want to do it for ulterior reasons. It's one of the most argued concepts in the fitness industry. I am goddamn sure that even the most fittest people do indulge in alcohol or have their own individual vices. When it's the right time, everybody has an escape.

What's the fuss about alcohol?

Alcohol also has calories. Not calories like carbohydrates which are converted into glucose. You see, simple terms, metabolism (absorption) of PCF, gives you energy. Metabolism of alcohol makes you drunk. Alcohol is not magic, its calories are not waived off. Alcohol is processed from food if you did not know. For the body, it is still data.

Knowing what alcohol contains what amount of calories and its PCF is the difference between you and the average binge drinker. You are not a geek. You are just better informed. Same goes for any vice, see how much you can know before you indulge in it.

The enemy remains not the vices in itself but the things surrounding it. Like sweeteners in alcohol, food that you are susceptible to eat under the influence. It's the environment and how your body reacts to it that makes you eat more.

I will not stress about the science and unwanted complications of giving into your vices. But practically, these things may not be abstained. It can optimised for your goals and lifestyle. Optimal is the key word.

6. Cheating:

There are two schools of thought on this. One which says that you should never have a cheat day. The other which says that you can incorporate this concept to live a full life. I for one am from the latter school of thought. This is a wonderful mechanism in a way. You can psychologically program your mind to enjoy great things in life. A guilt free cheat day or a cheat meal comes only if you know the nuances of macros and calorie counting, for if not, your definition of a cheat day is no different from a layman like Aunt Ruchi, which is a waste of calories. For them cheating is cheating, for real. But for those who have read this book, it is cheating to the outside world. A perfectly fine day or for you.

Rule 1 - It has to be isolated: Separate, dedicated, isolated the time or the cheat is must. It doesn't just happen impulsively but it is kept away for an occasion or an event or something special. You do not get to cheat on a whim or a fancy. You have to earn it. Keep it at bay, enjoy and get back to life as usual but do not mix and make that a part of your life. If you do not isolate it, it's more likely you will binge instead of cheat.

Rule 2 - It has to be pre-planned: It's a 100 percent better if you plan them so that you can work towards it and after it accordingly. Follow this like the bible. It may sound foolish but these are just things that you're doing to train your mind in the long run. You are doing this so that when you are 50 or 60 you don't repent having to eat your own birthday cake. Plan your days, your meals and your activity heading towards the cheat, if you have read this book well enough, probably you will create a small deficit in the days leading upto the cheat (maybe it's your sister's wedding). Maybe, just maybe, track the calories you ate on your cheat day?

Rule 3 - It has to be post planned and compensated: The same planning that went into approaching the cheat goes into coming out from it. No, I do not mean to tell you to whip yourself and do guilty workouts and abstain from food. I suggest you to follow FDL. Follow what you learnt about your body and how it reacts from reading the book. Just keep yourself accountable, you went into negative, try and get back to 0. Thats step 1.

Do these 3 and pretty soon, you can cheat and it would do zero internal (mental) and external (body) damage to you.

7.   Okay to Chase Vanity:

Listen, multiple people try to do things in the easiest or hardest or the most efficient manner. They prefer doing things right and according to the narrative set by society. They lose weight or turn a fitness corner by following the "rules". If you want to lose weight or if you want to become fitter if you want to get that jawline, those abs, etc it's not your fault. It is wired in humans to be better. If you want to get that girlfriend/boyfriend of yours and for that you want to shed a few kilos (or more), then by all means do it. Same goes if you are feeble thin and want to build a muscular structure. It's okay to chase vanity during these times as it is a calculated decision that only has an upside. Okay to want to have broad shoulders, it's okay to want to have big biceps, it's okay to want to look good in front of the mirror or want to look good naked. I will not shy away from the fact that I also took inspiration from vanity goals. So many folks I know and stories that I continuously hear are from people that only did it for vanity and for the better, it worked out for them. There is this one woman I know who is doing it purely to piss off her ex-husband. Another friend of mine is trying to get a six pack to land a girlfriend. (not that it matters, ask Michael)

Some people do it so that they can be less insecure. Again, the goals might be whatever, they change from person to person but the point is you get to the bottom of it. There is no loser here. I'm not advocating a malicious way of doing anything. Far from it. But realise that you have 1 life. You'll lose out if you go "by the book". I am suggesting that there is quite literally nothing for anybody to lose.

Pick your motivation and go for it.

8. Concept of Rest

Rest is important, both for the mind and the body. Don't get me wrong, your goal has to be to consistently train your body for approximately 4 to 5 days or even 6 days (if your intensity is lower). But having a rest day or two is paramount. Rest helps in recovery, he is a huge factor in the muscle building process and, most of all, never lets you over exhaust. Which is not optimal. Not long-term sustainable. Moderation is key. Otherwise, where is the fun in this? This training thing somehow has to become a part of your life just like all your take a poop, eat lunch, have a shower. Plan your rest days, your rest time, etc. Make sure you deserve them, make sure that you consider them to be as important as a normal day. This helps you stay sane.

9.   Over Eating, Pleasure Eating Comfort Food:

Here are a few scenarios that piss fit people off!

"I had a very tough day so I'm going to order pizza and lie down on the couch."

"I just broke up with my boyfriend so I am going to dig into the tub of ice cream. (why the heck do you have an ice cream tub in the freezer?)"

"I feel absolutely bored so let me go check what's in the fridge."

Eating without reason, eating due to emotional impulses, eating because you are bored is one of the worst things that you could do. So many of us are guilty of it. It really boils down to how you psychologically perceive eating. If you have ever come across Pavlov's Classical conditioning theory, you would know. Your habit of eating emotional responses will make it a very tough habit to break. Emotional eating has to stop, pointless eating adds extra calories to your day that simply does not add any value. It only leads you to eating more the next time that you are faced with that situation. For example maybe you have another break up or maybe you have another tough day, this thing does not stop. Every single thing goes down the drain because of one day's mischievousness. This eating mostly involves what millennials call "comfort food". Do not stock food at home and hoard them if you don't need it. Come on, go out and get these comfort foods if need be but just don't fall into the habit of mindless eating without reason. This habit falls in the bucket of one of the toughest habits to break. Tame your mind over time and hold yourself accountable. Do not lose battles with a non-living thing - food.

10.   Social Pressure:

Humans are social beings. You would not believe it but peer pressure can significantly affect your fitness life. Even the most independent, self-reliant person will fall to social pressure. These are usually your thin friends, your metabolically gifted friends or your "don't care about Fitness" friend. Social pressures exist.

Maybe they pressure you for another drink, maybe you guys are hanging out and you are having a salad while they are having something really appetizing, they ask you to take a bite.

Maybe you're saving your calories for something special for the night and in the afternoon your friends force you or mock you for making a cleverer macro choice. Don't unfriend them, that's stupid advice. But change your perspective (as you certainly cannot theirs), take it on the chin. Take this from me, they will be inspired by you later. When they turn out to be aunt Ruchis of the world and you walk super fit at 70 years of age. This is your grind. Do not ever refrain from pointing out the obvious. There is nothing wrong in accepting that you are following an eating pattern or dieting or making some changes and that is for your good only. These mocks or emotional blackmails that your best friends, family, peers may throw upon you are highly short-term.

It is a rule of thumb when it comes to eating and drinking that you will never, ever fall for or succumb to anybody's pressure even if it means your own goddamn wedding for that matter. You are not flowing with the flow. You do you.

11. Portion Control:

This is an extension to the point of over-eating. Not only has the quantum of calorie intake increased over time, it has also led to an increase in the size of servings, portions, spoons, pours and the bites. These are the droplets of water that make up the pond. The pond being your body. So, the next time when you subconsciously take that extra serving or that bite, remember, each and every calorie matters. I am not asking you to abstain, but yes get yourself used to a little bit lesser. The body can do with a bit lesser. It can get used to less if you feed it less. Else, it will keep asking for more.

Practice it, whenever you are eating just think about the serving size, always. Weigh it in your mind. Approximate the PCF and see if it's worth it. This applies to the number of Rotis/Dosas/Idlis, amount of curry, the length of your order at the restaurant and so on.

This also gives you the opportunity to mix up and add more calories of a different variety. Let us assume that you are on a cheat day at a family get together. Other than having just two portions of each dish which adds up to 600 g of food. You can get 4/6/8 dishes of lesser portions adding up to the same. Again, strictly assuming here that we are not counting macros. Less is okay. More is not okay. There's always more out there to eat next time.

Portion control does not mean eating mini calorie bombs spread across the whole day.

No, this habit of yours probably adds up to about 3000+ cal at the end of the day. That does not work. Portion control is for you to strictly stay cognisant of the quantum of calories going as intake. If I can summarise this point I would say, macros matter yes, but they go out of the window if you are just eating too damn much. That will by default put you in a surplus.

12.   A Tip for Women - Make Weights Your Best Friends.

Strength training, a step ahead of just resistance training, is not just for men. This is highly misconstrued by modern society. My strong advice to women would be to do strength training. Lift weights. If it were a tough thing to gain muscle for men, because of your hormonal differences, it becomes even tougher for women to gain muscle. Whatever they do gain thanks to strength training really gives the body a proper shape and structure. Through the idea that women who lift weights become bulky/manly out of the window. You don't just balloon up because you lift weights or do any sort of resistance training. There are no men and women exercises. The efficacy of the exercise is different because we are different by nature. If you have ever come across a really fit girl and you have no idea about training or you didn't read this book, most would consider that she does yoga or running or stereotype her instantly. Believe me the chances are high that she does some or the other sort of resistance training with the weights being in the mix. Go on, ask, question, research about the fittest girl you know and just enquire if weight training is a part of her regime or not. For girls, it is much more of a blessing than for a boy. The results of resistance training mainly old school weightlifting on them is amazing in terms of body composition and structure. I can say, that from a fitness point of view, most answers to most women's questions lies in weightlifting. Go on, go lift some weights.

13. Cravings

We all have cravings, everybody in the world has their fair share of guilty food pleasures. Thoughts from the left end of the fitness spectrum would be to completely avoid them and face going mad, this is long-term unsustainable. The other end of the spectrum would tell you to completely go bonkers, give into them, lose your small mental battles and repent gaining weight or losing progress when you see yourself in the mirror.

I have chosen an economic approach where you take ownership and are accountable for every time you crave something. It's not a problem if you fall for them here and there as this method takes care of it.

1. Water – Craving a cheesecake? Grab a full bottle of water, gulp it. The whole thing. Most cravings are actually not

because of hunger but because we want something in our system. Water is 83% of all cravings, don't go by that number, but believe in it, reinforce it, even though the numerical accuracy may be off, it does it's job.

2. Protein – Craving a pizza? Force-feed yourself (irrespective of where you stand in your daily calories) with chicken, eggs, broccoli. Satiation, something that you know by now. Just anything high in protein and fibre does its job. Once you are satiated, full stomach with this kind of food, it would almost be sickening to have anything else, believe me. Next time you're in this position do it for yourself, grab six boiled eggs and eat it and then ask yourself if you would have a pizza right after or not.

3. Track in advance – This has been common for most things. Track your food using an app or any other way in general when you are dieting. But, doing it in advance helps a lot. Tracking for tomorrow or, if you know that there is a party at the weekend, tracking and logging your food in advance. Log in what you must eat and only that. Once that is entered and locked in, it cannot change. This strongly prevents you from craving indulgence.

4. The selfie trick – Something that has worked so brilliantly would be my (if patentable) selfie trick. Every time you have that craving feeling, are about to succumb to that ice cream or doughnut or burger or anything under the Sun, grab a quick selfie of yours, if possible without clothes. Look at that selfie, ask yourself if that body you're seeing is okay or is that dish worth it? This did wonders for me, not only did it change my attention but it also, more often than not, it worked. Now this seems extreme but these are the steps, sacrifices that one takes to achieve freedom.

Introspect, ask yourself all possible questions. I had an album of photos at the end of the whole last year in my gallery that surpassed 300+ images of myself in places ranging from the home to a flight to clubs to restaurants.

There's no losing in this battle, either you enjoyed your indulgence or you won a small mental battle with your mind. The selfie trick is a real bonus, it keeps track of all the times you've felt this feeling and enumerates the times you've won or lost.

14.   A Different Kind of Self-Love!

Screw body positivity and the plus size movement. No seriously. I was a huge advocate for it once and I feel sick. Do yourself and your body a favor and show it some love by treating it right, feeding it right and training it right. Sometimes, the majority of your look is how you take care of your "self" in general. Your grooming, skin care and dressing habits and the like. It just shows if somebody loves themselves. Not their egotistic loving themselves, but care for the body that god has given them. Train your mind to care about, what we have forgotten arc general concepts like grooming, hitting the gym, eating right and dressing. These things go a long way. Being comfortable in your own skin IS NOT EQUAL TO ACCEPTING THE STATUS QUO! There is no rocket science in this. Fit people are considered to be a bit more attractive than fat people. Likewise, well dressed and well-groomed people are naturally considered attractive than the opposite ones. We can't rewire society but you can rewire yourself.

15.   Avoid the Short Cuts. PERIOD!!!

Coach your mind, tell it, practice it and do whatever you can to avoid taking short cuts. Stop going for the fix, the easier way out, the hack, the tip, the magic pill. If your pillars and foundation aren't strong, your micro-optimisation of a few things here and there will help you to no end. I mean things like weight loss teas, meal replacements, steroids, new age fake supplements that you have not researched. I had to address this point having done enough research and being a part of the food industry in general.

There is more than a good enough chance that the favourite physique on social media or that favourite actor that got that body used steroids. There is more than a good enough chance that a new revolutionary product that is marketed to you is fake, pseudo-science backed meant to make a quick buck. Don't get me wrong, amazing, revolutionary products exist. Things that have changed the industry but for the most part, hard work takes time. Products act as aid, that is it. Supplements and shortcuts should be to smoothen the edges not make the sculpture in the first place. Know that there are substances are synthetic (man made) that can accelerate fitness results, be it muscle gain or fat loss. People also inject or consume human produced hormones like testosterone and hGH that mimic the effects of that of steroids. Steroids are more common in the industry than you think. Likewise there are a million short cut ways to "get there" ranging from medications to surgeries and what not. There is a synthetic alternative to almost everything natural. Do yourself a long term favour, stay away from short cuts in your fitness life.

BONUS TIP:

Being part of movements?

How to know if what you're doing is right or wrong? Ask yourself, does what I am buying into, resemble a cult?

Always make way for something that is science and logic based.

I do not want to complicate things and throw garbage in your brain. There is more than a trick or two that is being played on you by the free market sources in the food and fitness industry. They don't go "market first" but they go "product first". Hey, detoxing is catching on, boom here is the solution. "Detox Tea". Nutritionally educated people are propping up - boom, "superfoods" (whatever that means). People are studying micronutrients - boom "vitamin supplements".

Here's a thought for the road. Your body detoxes itself, learn the underlying concept of macronutrients and micronutrients, be sane, that is your superfood. Learn and educate yourself about metabolism, be curious, that will do more good than non-prescribed supplements that they recommend "you must take" can. Do yourselves and others a favour separate the sound from the noise when it comes to what is marketed to you.

There is a reason why this is a book and not a demonstration, why I have chosen to concentrate on theory and not the practical approach. Exercises, science, diets, even tricks are things that can be brute forced to you. I sincerely believe that food and fitness, eating and activity, intake and exercise, whatever you term them as, (the 2 pillars of this book) as are mental battles first. It is a very strange fact that the mind has control and say as to how our body looks. But once that is conquered, either by brute forcing it or by expanding our knowledge or by introspecting it or sometimes just by being aware of it, it does wonders. I sincerely hope you all win your mental battles when it comes to fitness.

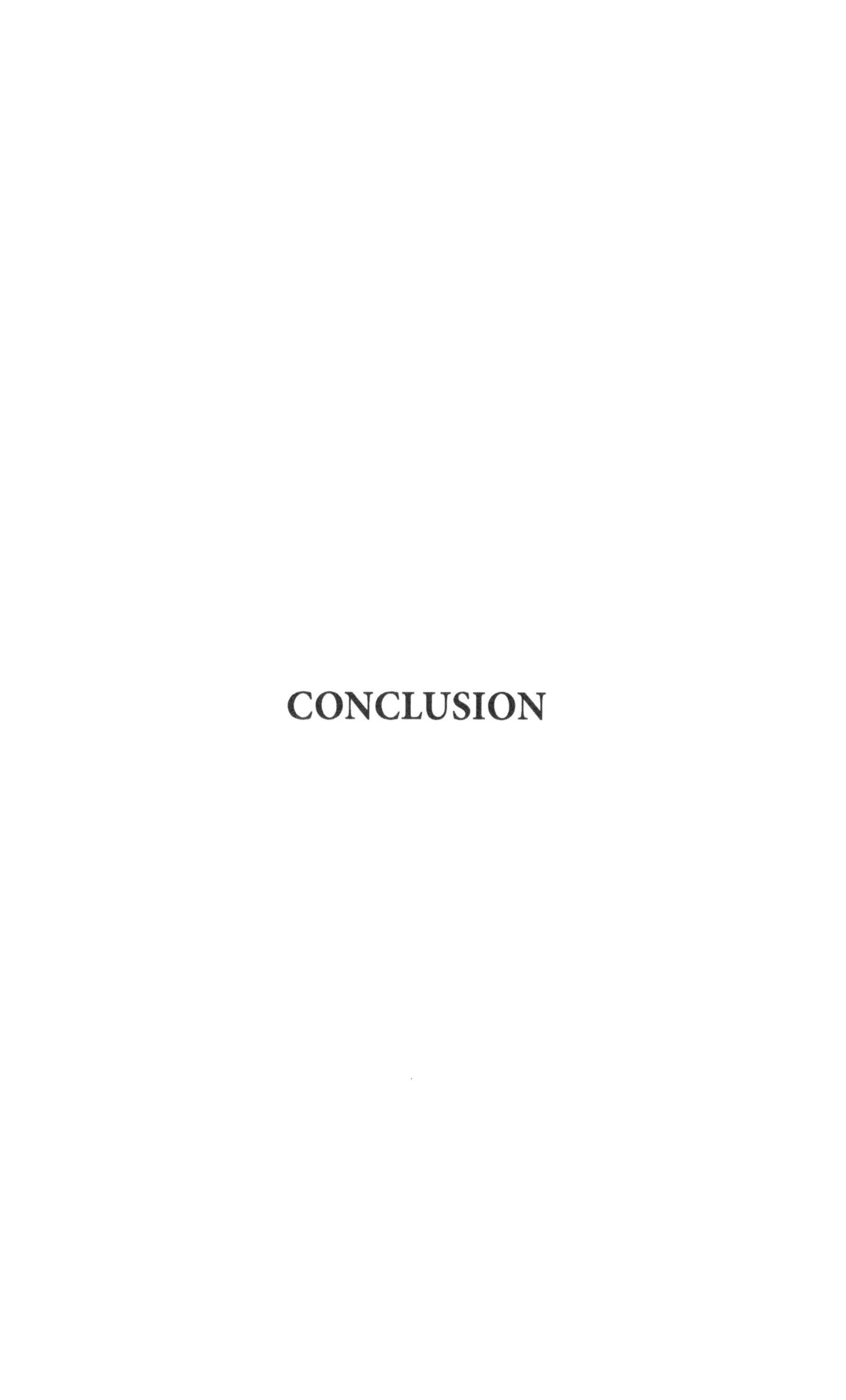

CONCLUSION

Here is what I will leave with you,

Your goal is Fitness and Nutritional freedom. To get there; (I assume you must have encountered these words more than often in the book)

- Think long term sustenance.

- Question every darn thing. Don't go with the flow.

- Build from scratch. Pillars, fundamentals, then tricks.

- Do the smart work hard.

- Remember the models - Food Quotient/Activity Quotient/ The Big 4/The Macro Math/The Weight Formula/The CYD/FDL/IIFYM/FTL/The Gym Commandments/Pain vs Exhaustion/The Psychological Tips plus whatever you gleaned from the book. These are just my fitness models. I'm sure over time, you will build your models too.

- Aim to be your own trainer, your own dietician, your own therapist and influencer. This is a part of life but not life itself.

Last but not the least,

Ask yourself, are you more like Aunt Ruchi, Kiara, Michael, My Dad or someone fudged in between? Therein lies the answer to where exactly you are and how far you have yet to go.

Go on, live a life of superpowers!

The End

www.ingramcontent.com/pod-product-compliance
Lightning Source LLC
Chambersburg PA
CBHW051051250726
48656CB00001B/251